# Pregnant & Lovin' It

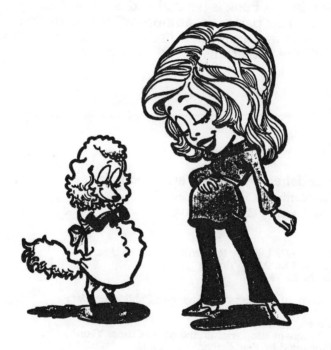

Lindsay R. Curtis, M.D.
Yvonne Coroles, R.N.

PRICE STERN SLOAN
Los Angeles

Notice: The information in this book is true and complete to the best of our knowledge. The book is intended only as an informative guide for those wishing to know more about pregnancy. In no way is this book intended to replace, countermand or conflict with the advice given to you by your doctor.

There are many variables to any illness or surgical condition. Your doctor knows your symptoms, signs, allergies, general health and the many other variables that challenge his/her judgment in caring for you as a patient.

The ultimate decision concerning any treatment should be made between you and your doctor, and we strongly recommend that you follow his/her advice. The information in this book is general and is offered with no guarantees on the part of the authors or Price Stern Sloan, Inc. The authors and publisher disclaim all liability in connection with the use of this book.

**Published by Price Stern Sloan, Inc.**
360 North La Cienega Boulevard
Los Angeles, California 90048


©1985, 1977 Lindsay R. Curtis Printed in U.S.A.
Revised for 22nd Printing
27 26 25 24

Library of Congress Cataloging-in-Publication Data

Curtis, Lindsay R.
    Pregnant and lovin' it/Lindsay R. Curtis, Yvonne Coroles;
illustrated by Paul Farber.—Rev. ed.
        p.        cm.
    Includes index.
    ISBN 0-89586-763-X:
    1. Pregnancy—Miscellanea. 2.  2. Childbirth—Miscellanea.
I. Coroles, Yvonne.  II. Title
RG525.C94 1988
618.2'4—dc19

# TABLE OF CONTENTS

Purpose of This Book ............................................ **4**

**1** It Has to Start Somewhere ................................. **5**

**2** What Happens Next? ...................................... **13**

**3** Pregnancy Is Three Times Three ....................... **31**

**4** Prenatal Care—You're on Your Way! ................. **41**

**5** Nausea and Vomiting During Pregnancy ........... **51**

**6** Medicines in Pregnancy ................................. **57**

**7** What May I Do? .......................................... **63**

**8** The Rh-Factor ............................................ **69**

**9** Rubella (German Measles) During Pregnancy ...... **77**

**10** Husbands and Pregnancy .............................. **83**

**11** Danger Signs of Pregnancy ........................... **89**

**12** Some Normal Discomforts of Pregnancy ........... **95**

**13** Common Sexual Infections and Diseases ........... **99**

**14** Miscarriage and Labor That Starts too Early ....... **107**

**15** Bleeding Late in Pregnancy .......................... **114**

**16** Tubal Pregnancy—The Displaced Person ......... **117**

**17** What Is Toxemia of Pregnancy? ..................... **121**

**18** More Than One! ........................................ **125**

**19** X-Ray and Ultrasound ................................. **129**

**20** Cesarean Births ......................................... **133**

**21** Weight and See .......................................... **137**

**22** How Do I Know When to Go and What to Do? . **143**

**23** Delivery—So This Is How It Is! ..................... **155**

**24** Afterbirth—You Mean There's More? .............. **161**

**25** About Nursing . . . ..................................... **164**

**26** Come as You Are—The Baby That Is ............... **181**

**27** After My Baby, Then What? .......................... **185**

**28** Emergency Childbirth .................................. **196**

**29** Miscellaneous Questions .............................. **203**

**30** Contraception ........................................... **209**

Authors' Biographies .................................... **224**

Index ...................................................... **225**

# PURPOSE OF THIS BOOK

You are about to experience one of the greatest, most pleasurable events of your life. Giving birth to a baby is exciting and can be very rewarding. Much of the joy of having a baby is anticipation. For pregnancy to be joyful, you must be free of fear and full of confidence.

The purpose of this book is to answer common questions that arise in pregnancy. It is not intended to be encyclopedic. If we can answer your questions and set your mind at ease, our purpose will have been accomplished.

If you want to know the questions that trouble pregnant women, ask a woman who is pregnant. About 2,000 couples pass through our Childbirth Education Classes each year. In each of the eight lectures and demonstrations, they are encouraged to ask questions.

This book is the result of sifting and sorting through the many questions asked and selecting the most common ones. We hope you will find the answer to your questions among them.

Artist Paul Farber has followed our mother-to-be, along with her pet poodle, through many of the trials and triumphs of pregnancy. We hope you will find the illustrations entertaining and informative.

*Note:* In this book we use the masculine pronoun "he" when referring to the baby. This in no way reflects a preference for either sex.

# 1.

## IT HAS TO START SOMEWHERE!

1. *How soon should I go to the doctor?*

Some doctors want to see you after you have missed two menstrual periods. It's difficult to tell for certain about pregnancy if you are examined too soon after missing your first menstrual period.

Many women become anxious and nervous if they go two weeks over their period. If you are anxious about your condition, phone your doctor and he may see you sooner.

2. *How early will my pregnancy test be positive?*

There is a pregnancy test performed with a sample of your urine or blood that is 95 to 98% reliable. It can confirm pregnancy even a few days after conception. Usually it isn't necessary to know that soon.

A pregnancy test is not performed routinely unless there is some compelling reason. The doctor can usually rely on his clinical findings to determine if you are pregnant.

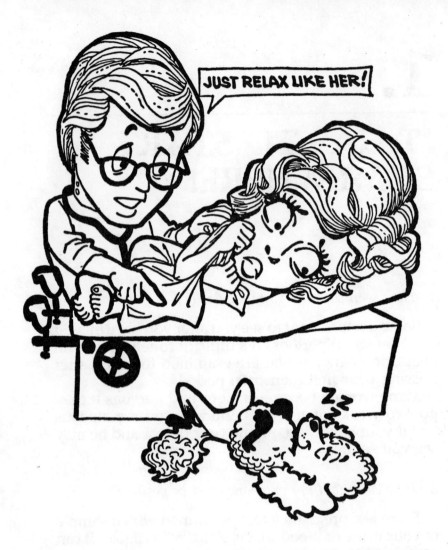

*I've never had a pelvic examination. What should I expect?*

3. *Other than missing a menstrual period, what are other early signs of pregnancy?*

Don't rely completely on a missed menstrual period because it isn't always dependable. In addition to missing a menstrual period you may notice:
- Morning sickness.
- Engorgement and soreness of your breasts.
- Easy fatigue.
- Frequent urination. You may also have to get up in the middle of the night to urinate.
- Dark discoloration of the skin in the disk around your nipples.
- Anxiety. This varies with the individual.

These signs and symptoms vary with each expectant mother. Other symptoms may be observed as pregnancy progresses.

4. *I've never had a pelvic examination. What should I expect?*

A pelvic examination is only part of a complete gynecological examination. Your doctor will also examine your head, neck, heart, lungs, breasts, abdomen, arms and legs.

In a pelvic examination, you must lie on your back on a special examination table. Knees are drawn up, and your feet are in stirrups. This allows the doctor to conveniently check your female organs. It helps to take a deep breath, then slowly let it out for 10 counts. This will help you relax.

After he inserts an instrument called a *speculum* into your vagina, he can look at the cervix (the mouth of the uterus) and take a pap smear. He can also see if the cervix has undergone the typical changes of pregnancy. In pregnancy, the cervix changes from pink to blue and becomes softer.

With two fingers in the vagina, and his other hand on the abdomen, he makes a pelvic examination. If you take a deep breath, it will help you relax and make it easier for the doctor to outline your uterus, Fallopian tubes and ovaries. If your abdomen is relaxed, the doctor can detect the softening changes of pregnancy in these tissues, as well as any abnormalities, such as cysts or tumors.

Sometimes your doctor may wish to confirm the diagnosis of pregnancy with a pregnancy urine test. This test can be performed in his office in a few minutes.

5. *I have a friend who had all the symptoms of pregnancy, but she wasn't pregnant. Is this possible?*

This is called *false pregnancy* and may be found in women who greatly desire pregnancy but cannot conceive. It may also be found sometimes in women who fear pregnancy.

False pregnancy may cause vomiting, missed menstrual periods, weight gain and even *quickening*, feeling life. Unfortunately these women eventually realize they are not pregnant.

Normal women, under certain circumstances, experience the same sensations and symptoms. There is no explanation for many of these cases.

6. *I've always wondered where and how fertilization of the egg takes place.*

Sperm from the male are deposited in the vagina by intercourse. From this point, the sperm swim by means of their tails through the secretions of the vagina, making their way into the cervix.

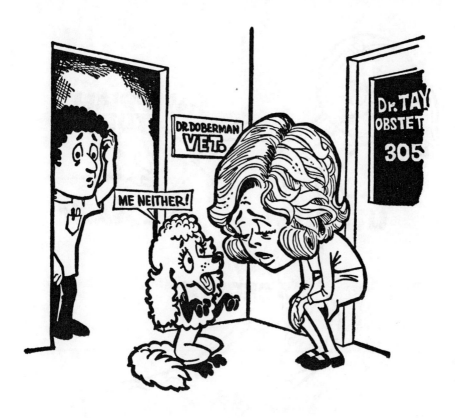

*I have a friend who had all the symptoms of pregnancy, but she wasn't pregnant. Is this possible?*

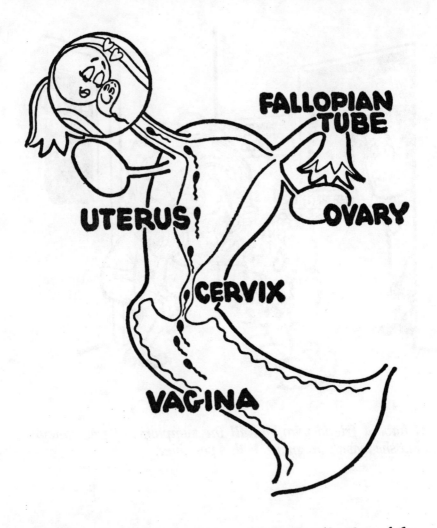

*I've always wondered where and how fertilization of the egg takes place.*

Swimming through the secretions found on the lining of the uterus, the sperm make their way into the Fallopian tube. In the outer part of the Fallopian tube, farthest from the uterus, the sperm meets the egg. Although several sperm may find their way into the tube, only one sperm penetrates the egg and fertilizes it.

The fertilized egg makes its way down the tube—it takes about three days—into the cavity of the uterus. In the meantime, the fertilized egg has already divided several times and has become a round ball of cells.

After four or five days in the uterine cavity, the fertilized egg becomes embedded in the nutritious lining of the uterine cavity. The egg begins to develop into an embryo, then into a fetus and finally into a full-term, fully developed baby, ready for birth.

7. *How long does a sperm remain alive after it has been deposited in the vagina?*

We are not absolutely sure. We think a sperm is capable of fertilization for two days. Sperm may remain active, but immobile, for a longer period than this.

Sperm require a lower-than-normal body temperature to survive. This may be the reason testicles are on the outside of the male body.

8. *How long does an egg remain alive after it is released from the ovary?*

We *think* it remains alive for 12 to 24 hours, then it dies and is discarded. Fertilization often takes place within 12 hours of ovulation.

Some researchers believe the fertile period in the female, the time during which she can conceive, is less than 12 hours. However, there are additional factors that may influence fertility.

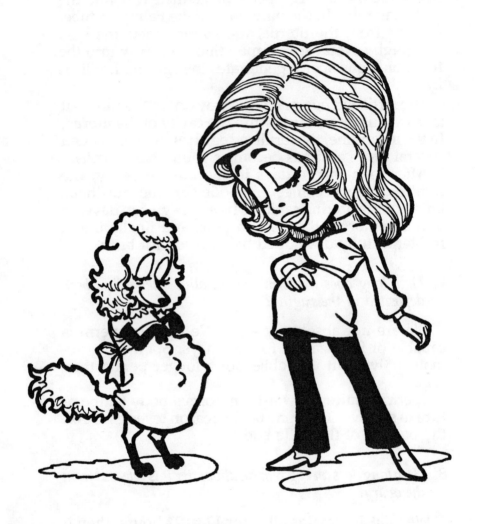

*What happens next?*

# 2.

# WHAT HAPPENS NEXT?

From the moment of conception you begin to change physically and emotionally. These changes vary with each individual. Let's discuss a few of them.

### 1. *Why are my breasts so tender?*

One of the first signs of pregnancy is tenderness and tingling of the breasts. Breasts feel full and become larger and more tender. This is because Nature, by means of hormones, is preparing your breasts for breast-feeding.

Whether you are going to breast-feed or not, your breasts are preparing for nursing. Engorgement, or fullness, in the breast of a pregnant woman is usually caused by a greater flow of blood, as well as an increase in the number and size of glands.

**2.** *Is it normal to have secretion from my nipples?*

Yes. The milky secretion is similar to *colostrum*, a watery fluid that is the forerunner of breast milk produced after the baby is born. Colostrum is good for the baby, although it may be a nuisance to you.

Secretion can often be controlled by inserting pads in your bra to absorb fluid. If leakage is excessive, a tiny plastic dish-cover, filled with paper tissue, can be worn inside the bra to keep your clothes dry.

**3.** *Why do birth-control pills, taken prior to pregnancy, foul up due dates?*

Occasionally you may miss one or several menstrual periods when you discontinue birth-control pills. For instance, you usually have a menstrual period within a couple of days after discontinuing the pill. But if you do not resume taking birth-control pills, you may fail to have another period for several months. This is the exception, not the rule.

Often cycles of women who have stopped taking birth-control pills are *anovulatory*, which means no egg is released from the ovary. When ovulation resumes, you become fertile and may become pregnant. After ovulating, you resume your menstrual period unless you are pregnant. When you do get pregnant, it may be difficult for you to know exactly when to calculate when the baby is due. This is the reason many doctors suggest waiting a few cycles before attempting pregnancy.

**4.** *What is the bag of waters?*

The *amniotic sac* holds the fetus as it grows. The fluid it contains is called *amniotic fluid*. The amniotic cavity starts as a tiny sac of water. Eventually this bag completely surrounds the baby, providing a watery cushion against temperature change, injury, pressure or inflammation as the baby grows. The water also keeps the baby from rubbing against the walls of the uterus and gives the baby room to grow.

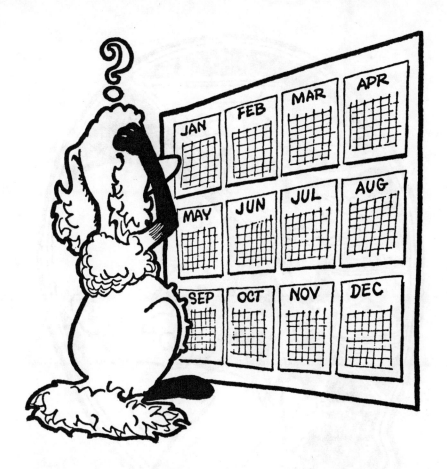

*Why do birth-control pills, taken prior to pregnancy, foul up due dates?*

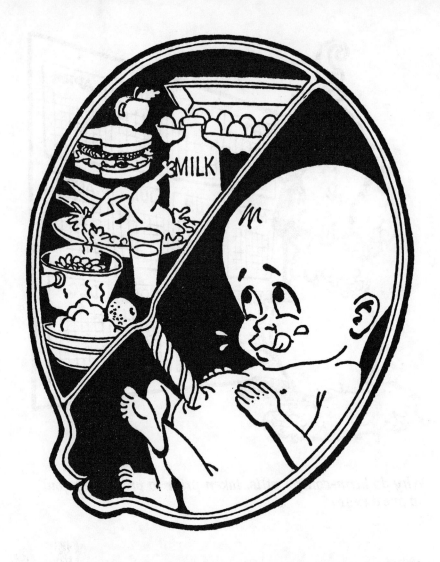

*If the baby is encased in water, how does he get food and how does he eliminate waste?*

## 5. *Where does the water come from?*

Amniotic fluid comes from your blood serum in the beginning. Later, as the baby develops, water comes from the fetus' urine. As the baby swallows amniotic fluid, his kidneys secrete urine into the amniotic fluid. The process continues as the fluid is recycled through the kidneys.

## 6. *Why do some women have more water than others?*

The average amount of water in the amniotic sac is a little over a quart. When this amount exceeds two quarts, it is abnormal and becomes uncomfortable for the mother. It can also place the baby at risk. Women may have only a tiny amount of water or a large amount. We do not know the reason. Too much (hydramnios) or too little (oligohydramnios) amniotic fluid may be a sign of fetal defect. Defects include spina bifida, where part of the covering of the brain or spinal cord is missing.

## 7. *If the baby is encased in water, how does he get food and how does he eliminate waste?*

Nourishment comes completely from you, through the placenta, into the baby's blood supply through the umbilical cord. Oxygen is also carried by the blood through the cord.

Urine from the fetus is eliminated into the amniotic fluid surrounding the baby. Waste in a fetus is minimal. It accumulates in the baby's bowel as a tarry, green-black material, called *meconium*. Normally, meconium is not eliminated from the bowel as a stool until after birth, unless the baby is subjected to stress or strain. Often stress occurs if the cord is compressed, causing the baby to struggle in his attempt to get oxygen.

## 8. *Does the baby produce urine before it is born?*

Yes, and it is secreted into the amniotic fluid.

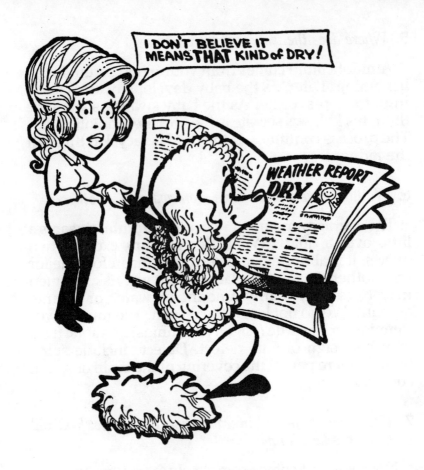

*What is a dry birth, and how dangerous it it?*

## 9. *Is it dangerous to have excessive water?*

There are certain complications for a mother-to-be with excessive water. More defective babies are born when there is more than the normal amount of amniotic fluid.

When there is excessive water, there is greater likelihood the bag of waters will break with a gush before labor begins. If this happens, the umbilical cord may wash past the baby and into the vagina. With subsequent labor contractions, the blood vessels in the cord become compressed between the baby's head and the cervix or pelvic wall.

Unless this compression is relieved and blood allowed to flow through the umbilical cord, the baby will suffocate. Sometimes the baby can be saved only by immediate delivery, which may require a Cesarean operation.

## 10. *What is a dry birth, and how dangerous is it?*

A true *dry* birth is almost non-existent. Amniotic fluid is secreted continuously, mostly by the baby's kidneys. It is not uncommon after the bag of waters breaks to have a great gush of amniotic fluid.

One purpose of this fluid is to lubricate the birth canal for passage of the baby. Because fluid continues to be formed, there is no such thing as a dry birth.

## 11. *What role does the afterbirth play in the development of the fetus?*

During its three-day journey down the tube to the uterine cavity, the fertilized egg divides many times. During the three or four days it remains in the uterine cavity, it continues to develop. By this time it needs more nourishment than uterine secretions can provide.

The embryo develops specialized cells on one side that enable it to burrow into the wall of the uterus. Here it establishes communication with your blood-

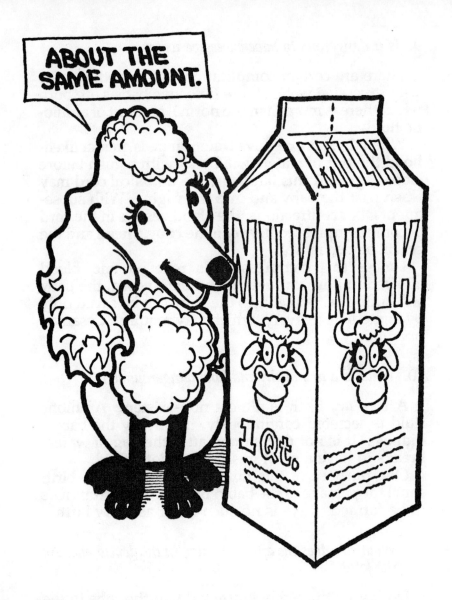

*The average amount of water in the amniotic sac is a little over a quart.*

stream. The specialized cells develop into the afterbirth, also known as the *placenta*.

The baby's blood and your blood never come in direct contact with each other. An exchange of oxygen and nourishment takes place between you through several layers of membranes in the placenta. The placenta serves as the middleman for this exchange. The placenta is also important in the production of hormones used by you and the fetus during pregnancy.

12. *Is there any way to estimate how large my baby might be at a given time in my pregnancy?*

Doctors use several methods that involve centimeters and lunar months, but these are hard to understand for most people. However, here a few simple rules to follow:

- One month—Half the size of the end of your little finger.
- Two months—As large as the end of your thumb.
- Three months—The size of your entire thumb.
- Four months—About the size of a hot dog.
- Five months—Weighs a little under a pound (460 grams) and is 10 inches long (26cm).
- Six months—Weighs about 1-1/2 pounds (700 grams) and is a little over 12 inches long (32cm).
- Seven months—Weighs 2-1/4 pounds (1kg) and is 15 inches long (38cm).
- Eight months—Weighs 4 to 5 pounds (1.8 to 2.3kg) and is 16 to 17 inches long (41 to 44cm).
- Nine months—Weighs 7 pounds (3.4kg) and is 21 inches long (54cm).

13. *Does a baby have normal digestion before birth?*

Yes, to a limited extent. However, a baby does not have bowel movements until after birth, unless asphyxia occurs, causing him to struggle or strain. Fecal material (meconium) produced before birth is retained in the intestinal tract. It looks like soft, black tar.

**14.** *Does my baby breathe while I am carrying him?*

Sort of. He does not breathe air, of course. But rhythmic respiratory movements may occur as early as 12 weeks and continue until birth. After he is born, the baby continues what he has been practicing.

**15.** *Do babies have hiccups?*

Babies have hiccups frequently before birth. It's a common reflex effect of the diaphragm. Some babies are more prone to this than others.

**16.** *What are the soft spots in the baby's head?*

These are called *fontanels,* and they mark the juncture of various bones of the baby's head. The bones are purposely unjoined before birth so they can "give" during delivery. They may even overlap each other, if necessary, as the baby's head is compressed when passing through the birth canal.

The soft spots have no significance except they withdraw if the baby becomes markedly dehydrated. The size of the soft spots is not important. Soft spots are also useful in determining fetal position by vaginal exam during delivery.

Fontanels usually close spontaneously as bones grow together and cover the spaces. This process is complete by about 18 months of age.

**17.** *Do boys weigh more at birth than girls?*

Yes. Boys usually weigh about 3 ounces (85 grams) more than girls.

**18.** *What is the purpose of the umbilical cord?*

The cord contains two arteries and one vein that connect the placenta and baby. The cord is surrounded by a jellylike material. The covering of the cord is a continuation of the amniotic sac.

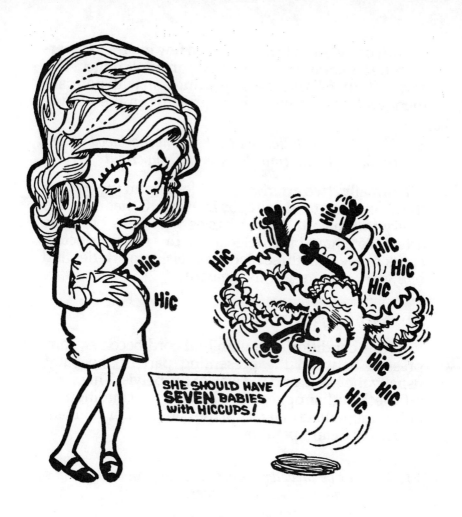

Do babies have hiccups?

The cord varies in length from a few inches to several feet. It is about the thickness of an adult finger. The cord is the baby's lifeline, supplying him with nourishment and oxygen while he is growing in the uterus.

19. *I have heard a doctor counts the number of blood vessels in the umbilical cord. Why is this important?*

Normally, two arteries carry blood from the baby to the placenta. About one baby in every 100 has only one artery in the cord. Of the babies who have only one artery, 25% have birth defects. For this reason, doctors check to see if all three blood vessels, two arteries and one vein, are present in the cord.

20. *What is a prolapsed cord?*

In this condition, the umbilical cord becomes compressed between the presenting part of the baby, usually the head, and the wall of the pelvis. This shuts off the blood supply to the baby. This condition requires immediate delivery of the baby, either vaginally or by Cesarean operation.

21. *Can sex be predetermined? Can we plan conception so we'll have one sex or the other?*

There is some evidence that indicates coitus at the exact time of ovulation, 14 days before the onset of the next menstrual period, is more likely to produce a boy. Coitus before this time is more likely to produce a girl. An alkaline precoital douche seems to be more favorable for production of a male and an acid douche for a female.

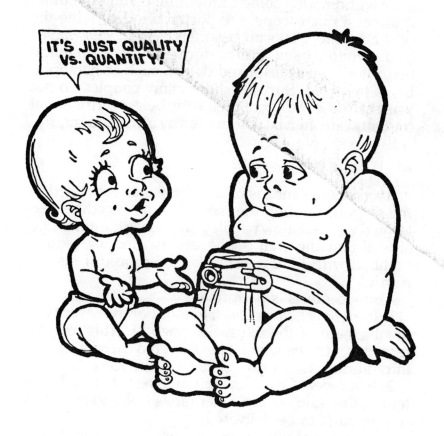

*Do boys weigh more than girls at birth?*

## 22. Can sex be determined before birth?

By withdrawing some amniotic fluid and examining it under a microscope, the doctor can determine the sex of the baby. This procedure is called *amniocentesis*. In determining sex, it is performed only for medical reasons where a sex-linked defect, such as hemophilia, is involved. Surveys show many couples do not want to know the sex of their baby before birth. Sex of the baby can often be determined by ultrasonography.

## 23. What is amniocentesis?

*Amniocentesis* means to tap the water contained in the sac surrounding the baby. It is a procedure performed with a hollow needle that pierces the abdominal wall and the wall of the uterus. Because skin is numbed with local anesthesia, the procedure is not painful.

Amniocentesis is performed:

1. In *erythroblastosis fetalis*, to monitor the severity of involvement of the fetus. See page 71. This test determines if the baby must be delivered early, given an intrauterine transfusion or needs other care.

2. In a repeat Cesarean section to test chemical content of the fluid, which determines if the baby is mature enough to be delivered.

3. In patients whose membranes have broken (the water sac has ruptured) to test fluid for evidence of infection. If there is no infection, the urgency of delivery is not as great. This is important in patients whose infants would be premature if they were delivered too early.

4. In most patients over 35 years old, to test for Down's Syndrome in the fetus.

## 24. *How fast does the fetus grow and develop?*

During the *first two weeks*, the egg divides rapidly. It soon becomes a ball of cells, with a large yolk sac for nutrition. This sphere of cells develops an amniotic sac that envelops the *embryo*. At this stage, the embryo and sac have a relationship similar to a fist pushed into a small balloon containing water. The part of the balloon over the fist develops into skin covering the fetus. The rest of the balloon becomes the amniotic sac.

In the *third week*, heart, brain and limb buds develop. A rudimentary tail is still present. In the *fourth week*, the embryo grows rapidly. The first traces of eyes, ears, nose and all other organs appear.

During the *second month*, 4 to 8 weeks, there is a marked growth of head size in proportion to body. The heart begins to beat and circulation begins. After 8 weeks, the embryo is called a *fetus*.

In the *third month*, 8 to 12 weeks, fingers and toes are recognizable with soft nails. The fetus begins to move. Sex organs begin to develop, but sex cannot be determined except by microscope.

In the *fourth month*, 12 to 16 weeks, sex is recognizable. The fetus is 4 to 6 inches long (10 to 15cm). The vagina and anus are open, and some digestion begins.

In the *fifth month*, 16 to 20 weeks, downy hair covers the body with slightly more on top of the head. Eyelids are still fused.

In the *sixth month*, 20 to 24 weeks, skin is thin, red and wrinkled, with some fat deposits under it. The head is still large compared to the body. If born, the baby will attempt to breathe and may survive with specialized care.

In the *seventh month*, 24 to 28 weeks, skin is covered with material called *vernix*. The covering membrane disappears from eyes, and eyelids separate. Sight and hearing are usually the last things to develop, but should be all right now. With modern, intensive newborn care, infants as early as 26 weeks are being delivered by Cesarean section and surviving. Long-term results are needed to evaluate the effects premature delivery has on ultimate development of the infant.

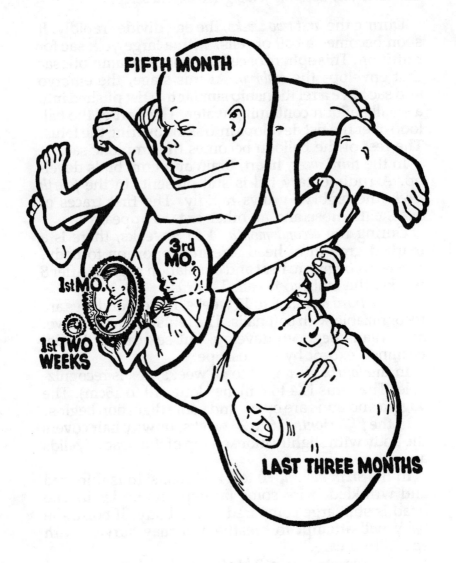

FIFTH MONTH

3rd MO.

1st MO.

1st TWO WEEKS

LAST THREE MONTHS

*Growth and development of the fetus.*

In the *eighth month,* 28 to 32 weeks, skin still looks wrinkled because of the lack of fat under it. At this point, the baby is still subject to *atelectasis,* a condition in which lungs are not mature enough to expand as they should. If born now, the baby is likely to survive with good care.

In the *ninth month,* 32 to 36 weeks, the face is no longer wrinkled. If born now, the baby should survive.

In the *tenth month,* 36 to 40 weeks, skin is smooth, without down, except over the shoulders. Hair is probably dark. The body is covered with vernix. Nails have grown beyond finger and toe tips. Testicles are in the scrotum in males. Lips of the vagina are developed and touch each other in the female. Skull bones are calcified. Eyes are slate-colored, but it is impossible to predict ultimate color.

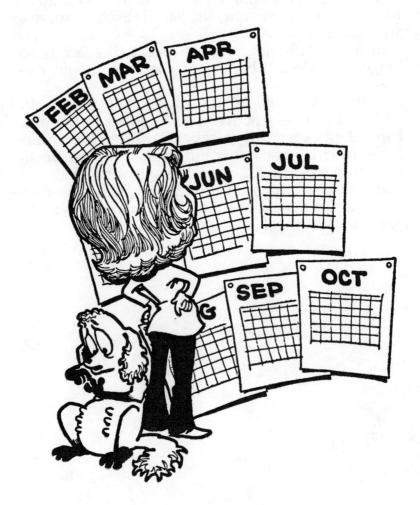

*How far along am I?*

# 3.

# PREGNANCY IS THREE TIMES THREE

The average pregnancy lasts about nine months. The time is divided into three sections of three months each, called the *first*, *second* and *third trimesters of pregnancy*.

Another way to calculate the duration of pregnancy is by lunar months, consisting of 28 days each. In this case, there are 10 lunar months of pregnancy: 28 days x 10 months = 280 days.

## 1. *How far along am I?*

Pregnancy takes 280 days, counting from the first day of your last menstrual period. This assumes a 28-day menstrual cycle in which ovulation and fertilization occur on the 14th day, counting from the first day of flow. The actual pregnancy lasts for about 266 days—280 minus 14.

A doctor usually counts from the first day of your last menstrual period, even though the pregnancy did not begin until two weeks later. If he says you are eight weeks pregnant, he means eight weeks from your last menstrual period, even though the embryo is only 6 weeks old.

Women tend to say, "I am in my fourth month." This is vague. It would be more accurate to say, "I am 12 weeks along." This assumes you are counting from the first day of your last menstrual period.

### 2. *When is my baby due?*

To calculate when your baby is due, most doctors count back three months from the first day of your last menstrual period and add seven days. For instance, if your last menstrual period began May 2nd, the baby is probably due February 9th.

It is not uncommon or abnormal to have your baby two weeks early or two weeks late. Only one woman in 10 delivers on the exact due date.

### 3. *Is there any way to keep my breasts this full after my baby?*

No. Many small-busted women have expressed this wish, but breast enlargement is due to temporary engorgement. With a good supportive bra, good posture and daily breast exercises, you may be able to maintain or build more desirable breasts.

### 4. *What are the small bumps around my nipples?*

These small glands in the disk around the nipple enlarge in pregnancy. They lubricate the area around the nipple, allowing for easier, less-painful nursing.

The appearance of these *tubercles*, as they are called, along with pigmentation of the disk surrounding the nipple, is an early sign of pregnancy.

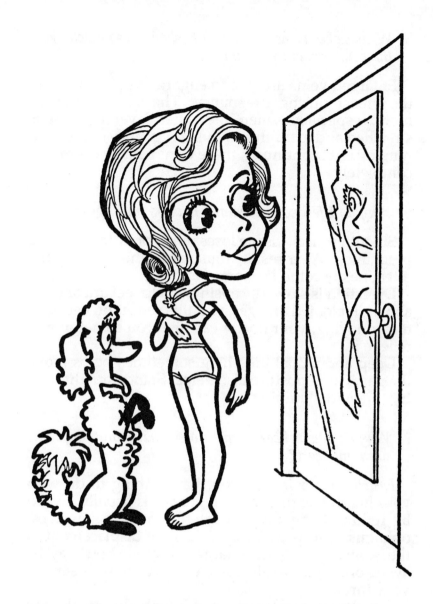

*Is there any way to keep my breasts this full after my baby?*

5. *What makes veins of my breasts show up so much? Will the veins remain permanently?*

Enlarged veins are due to engorgement of blood in the breast during pregnancy. The veins show up more, especially when the outer layer of skin is stretched and extra-thin. When pregnancy is over and nursing is discontinued, these veins usually disappear completely.

6. *Why do I feel so bloated and have so much gas?*

Smooth muscle tissue loses much of its tone during pregnancy. As a result, muscles in the walls of the intestines become lazy and flabby.

Digestion is slowed, causing you to feel uncomfortably full, bloated and gassy. If this sensation becomes too annoying, your doctor can give you something to relieve it.

Deep abdominal breathing sometimes helps move the gas. Good posture also helps. Stand straight, and try to avoid slumping.

7. *Why do I have heartburn? Does it have anything to do with my heart?*

*Heartburn,* or indigestion, has nothing to do with your heart. Heartburn in pregnancy is usually caused by reflux of the gastric contents into the lower esophagus. This is probably a result of displacement of the stomach by your enlarging uterus. You may be aware of a sense of fullness or even a burning feeling in your throat.

A tablespoon of cream a half-hour before meals may relieve this discomfort. If you need additional relief, a teaspoon of antacid after meals will often help. Check with your doctor before you take *any* medication.

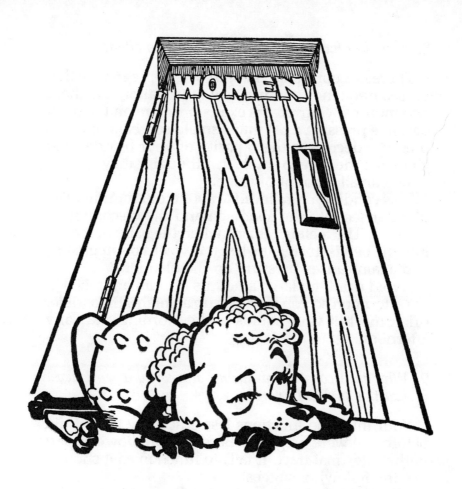

*Why do I have to go to the bathroom so often?*

## 8. Why do I have to go to the bathroom so often?

There is a hormonal change early in pregnancy that causes frequency and urgency of urination. At about two months, your uterus exerts pressure on the bladder, like pressing a fist into a small, soft balloon. This pressure decreases the capacity of your bladder and gives you the urge to empty it, although it may contain only a small amount of urine.

This condition is relieved at about four months. The uterus rises into the abdomen and the discomfort is relieved. The feeling returns when the baby descends into the pelvis during the last few weeks of pregnancy and again causes pressure on the bladder.

Avoid drinking large amounts of fluid after 4:00 in the afternoon so you won't be up all night. If possible, drink most of your liquids in the morning and early afternoon.

## 9. Why am I constipated during pregnancy when I never had this problem before?

Your intestine functions less efficiently than it did before you were pregnant. Because your bowel is part of the intestinal tract, it fails to function as it should. Try the following suggestions:

- Increase fluid intake, especially fruit juices.
- Develop regular bowel habits.
- Take only laxatives your doctor prescribes for you.
- Bulk-forming and stool-softening laxatives, such as Metamucil, may be preferable to more-irritating laxatives. Check with your doctor.
- A tablespoon of honey in half a glass of warm water helps some women.
- Place your feet up on a small stool while evacuating the bowel. Sitting up straight is less comfortable and often less effective.

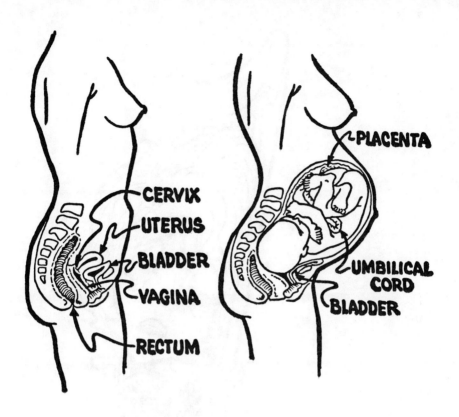

CERVIX
UTERUS
BLADDER
VAGINA
RECTUM

PLACENTA
UMBILICAL CORD
BLADDER

*Pressure from the uterus on the bladder causes you to urinate more than usual.*

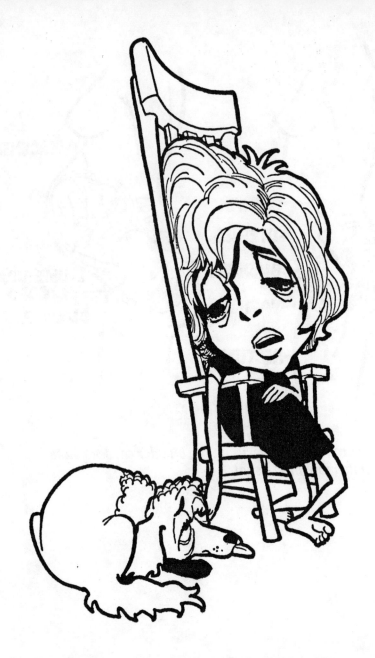

*Why am I so tired and need more sleep than usual?*

10. *Why do I cry so easily and become upset and angry over nothing?*

This mood change is due to hormonal changes. Pregnant women often become moody, depressed and easily upset. Under old English law, a pregnant woman's testimony was not acceptable in court because she was not considered reliable. This idea is exaggerated, but it shows the emotional change in pregnant women is not something new.

Most couples have a period of adjustment to make when they discover they are pregnant. Every couple does not become pregnant the exact moment they want to. Even if you have tried for years to have a baby, now that you're finally pregnant, you may wonder if you did the right thing.

You are not alone. Many women find their emotions are much more delicate during pregnancy. Be patient—you will return to normal with full control over your emotions when your pregnancy is over.

11. *Why am I so tired and need more sleep than usual?*

This may be due to a loss of muscle tone throughout your body. Fatigue is common in women who take birth-control pills, perhaps because the pill simulates pregnancy.

Sometimes it is Nature's way of slowing you down. With something as important as pregnancy going on in your body, you can't always continue the fast pace you set when you were not pregnant.

Fatigue is a temporary condition and may be expected to disappear when the pregnancy is over. In the meantime, get all the rest you can.

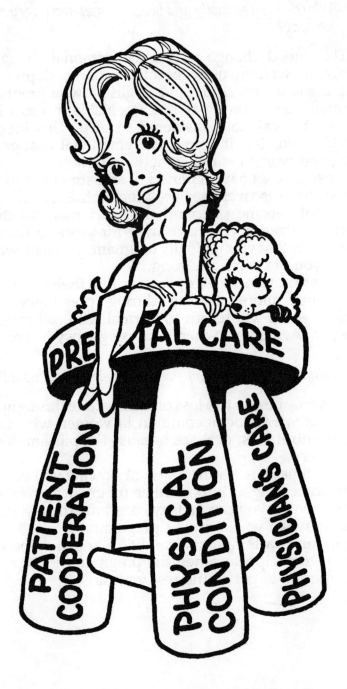

*Good prenatal care is like a three-legged stool.*

# 4.

# PRENATAL CARE— YOU'RE ON YOUR WAY!

Good prenatal care is like a three-legged stool, supported by your physician's care, your cooperation and your physical condition. Hopefully, all three will work together to make yours an enjoyable pregnancy.

We have already discussed your first pelvic examination. In addition to this, your doctor will check your heart, lungs, breasts and abdomen. He will do any other tests he thinks are necessary. He may want to check your pelvic measurements to see if your pelvis is large enough for a normal delivery.

He will weigh you, check your blood for Rh-factor and blood type and make sure you do not have a venereal disease. This latter test is required by law in most states. He will also test your blood to make sure you are not anemic and perform a routine check for the rubella antibody.

**1.** *Why must I give a urine specimen each time?*

The doctor checks your urine for sugar, to rule out diabetes, and for protein, to be sure kidneys are functioning normally. He also checks for bacteria or pus to make sure you don't have a urinary-tract infection.

**2.** *I never fainted before. Why should I during pregnancy?*

Fainting may be caused by the loss of tone in the muscle tissue that lines the blood vessels. Muscle tone is necessary to sustain blood pressure when the body position is changed.

If you take more time when you change positions, your body will adjust. You will be less likely to faint. Don't get up abruptly from a prone position. Roll to your side, then rise slowly.

If you feel like you're going to faint, sit down and place your head between your legs. Or lie down with your head lower than your body. If faintness still persists, have someone raise your legs higher than your body. This usually causes the blood to run to your head, and you will feel better almost immediately.

**3.** *Vision with my glasses seems different since I became pregnant. Do you think I should have my glasses checked?*

Some refraction changes occur normally in pregnancy. For this reason, a change in glasses won't solve the problem for long. To avoid eye strain, cut down on your reading, sewing, close-eye work and watching television.

Most headaches can be relieved by a mild analgesic or pain reliever prescribed by your doctor. If possible, put off getting new or different eyeglasses until after your pregnancy.

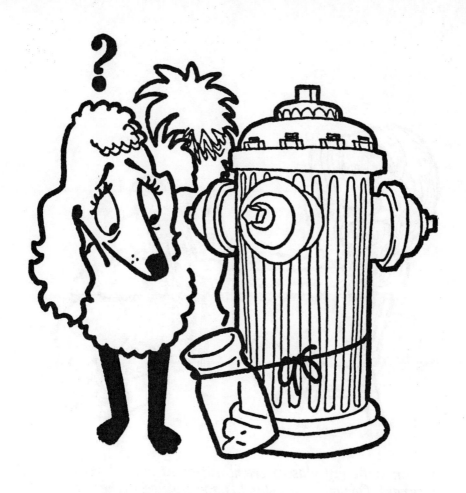

*Why must I give a urine specimen each time?*

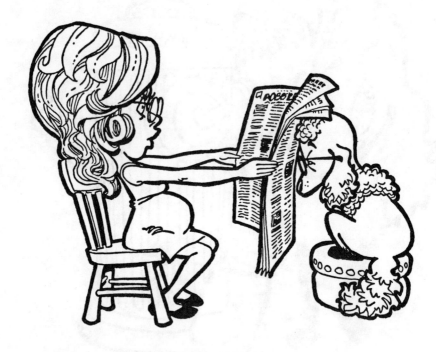

*Vision with my glasses seems different since I became pregnant. Do you think I should have my glasses checked?*

### 4. *What about drugs in pregnancy?*

Don't take *any* drugs during pregnancy without your doctor's permission. Avoid hormones, anti-thyroid drugs and streptomycin. Streptomycin may cause hearing loss in the baby.

Tetracycline may cause discoloration of the infant's teeth. Anticoagulants, given for phlebitis, may cause hemorrhaging in the mother if given too close to delivery time.

For additional information on drugs and pregnancy, see the section *Medicines in Pregnancy*, beginning on page 57.

### 5. *Is abdominal pain more serious in pregnancy?*

Even if you are pregnant, you can still have appendicitis, gall bladder attacks or other non-pregnancy-related problems. If in doubt about abdominal pain, call your doctor.

Be aware, but not alarmed, if your abdomen becomes firm or if you experience more than ordinary discomfort. This could indicate labor. If in doubt, notify your doctor!

### 6. *What is safe to use for constipation in pregnancy?*

This depends on how severe constipation is. There are a few simple things you may want to try. For example, drink at least two quarts of water a day. Certain fruits, such as prunes, raisins, apricots or other dried fruits, may help. Fruit juices may be effective.

Avoid harsh laxatives. Bulk laxatives or stool softeners, such as Metamucil, are better than stronger laxatives. However, these cannot function unless taken with a large amount of water. Don't take anything for constipation unless your doctor tells you to.

One or two tablespoons of honey in a glass of warm water may help. This remedy carries none of the disadvantages of laxatives.

## 7. *What can I do for backache in pregnancy?*

A firm mattress may help, along with a heating pad and a back massage by your husband. Try better posture habits, such as standing erect with weight evenly distributed on each foot. Some people stand on one foot, then the other. Flexing knees while standing also helps.

While sitting, you may find a straight-back chair is comfortable. To keep from slumping, tuck a small pillow at the small of your back. If your knees are lower than your hips when you sit, elevate your feet by using a foot stool or stack of books.

While lying on your back, place a pillow or folded blanket under your knees, under your abdomen or along your back. If you need to get something on the floor, squat down. This allows your legs to do the work, instead of putting strain on your back.

Exercise may also help relieve backache. But before you start any exercise program, check with your doctor.

## 8. *What can I do for cramps in my legs?*

Calcium and vitamin D help, as well as mild tranquilizers, especially if cramps occur at night.

Leg cramps and charley horses at night may be caused by pointing toes outward when you move or turn over. Use the reverse maneuver to rid yourself of the cramp. Bring your toes toward your face and push out your heels.

One or two tablespoons of honey in a glass of warm water may help. Some people think it acts as a muscle relaxant and mild sedative. Though the effect may be psychological, it may be worth trying and is not harmful.

A warm, not hot, bath is also relaxing before you retire.

## 9. *What about diet in pregnancy?*

A sample diet follows, and a discussion of some

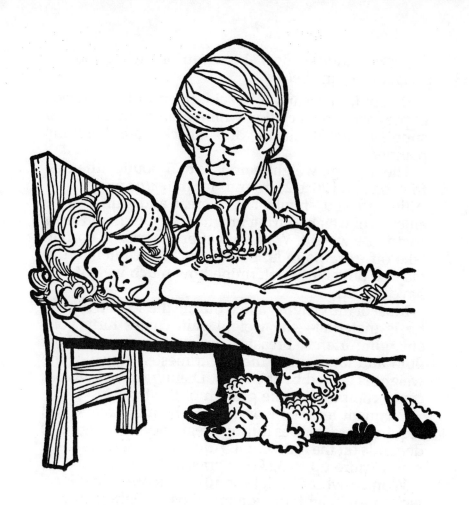

*What can I do for backache in pregnancy?*

things you should know about nutrition while you are pregnant begins below.

Except for iron and folic acid, the nutritional needs of pregnant and lactating women can be met without supplements if meals and snacks are carefully planned.

The average weight gain is 2 to 5 pounds the first trimester and 20 to 25 pounds for the *entire* pregnancy. Although you should not overeat and gain a large amount of weight during pregnancy, you should *never* try to lose weight. Wait until after the baby is born to take off extra pounds. Because of water retention, it may be difficult to determine how much weight you have gained.

Most of the weight gained during the second trimester is maternal—the weight gain comes form your enlarging uterus, breasts, blood, placenta, amniotic fluid and fat. During the last trimester, much of the weight is gained by the fetus. Dieting for weight loss could compromise the growth of the fetus.

Pregnant teenage women may be more active and require more calories during pregnancy, although this depends on the individual. Adolescent mothers-to-be may require up to 3,500 calories a day.

Women whose weight is 10% or more below ideal weight for height, or women whose weight gain during pregnancy is less than 2-1/2 pounds a month, may deliver low-birth-weight infants.

10. *What is a good diet to follow?*

An intake of about 2,500 calories per day is adequate for the average woman. Try to eat the following foods: **Protein**—Protein builds muscle tissue and skin. Protein is found in fish, chicken, meat, cheese and other dairy products, eggs, whole-grain cereals, beans and peas. At least 85 grams of protein daily is desirable.

**Carbohydrates**—Contrary to common belief, complex carbohydrates, such as bread and potatoes, are excellent foods to eat. They are not fattening unless garnished with large amounts of butter, jam, jelly, peanut butter or other high-calorie foods. Replace french-fried potatoes with a baked potato.

**Fats**—Fats are energy foods and contain certain vitamins you need. But they are also high in calories. Eat fats sparingly.

**Minerals**—Minerals are necessary for the baby's growth. Calcium and phosphorus are used by the fetus for bone growth and development. A quart of milk a day ensures an adequate amount of these minerals. Iron and folic acid are easier to take as tablets or capsules. It may be difficult to eat many iron-rich foods. Iodine requirements can be met by eating one seafood per week.

**Vitamins**—Vitamins can be supplied by one prenatal multivitamin capsule per day.

---

### SAMPLE DIET

**Breakfast**
4 ounces orange juice
1/2 cup oatmeal
1 slice toast
1 teaspoon butter
1 egg
8 ounces milk

**Lunch**
2 ounces cheese
2 slices bread
1 teaspoon butter
Salad of tomato and lettuce
8 ounces milk
1/2 grapefruit

**Dinner**
3 ounces lean meat, poultry or fish
1 medium potato, baked
1/2 cup carrots
2 teaspoons butter
1 medium apple

---

# PROTEIN AND CALORIE CONTENT OF SOME FOODS

| | Approximate Size of Portion | Approx. Protein (grams) | Calories |
|---|---|---|---|
| **Dairy Foods** | | | |
| Milk | | | |
| whole | 8 ounces | 9 | 160 |
| skimmed | 8 ounces | 9 | 90 |
| Cheese | | | |
| American | 1 slice | 8 | 110 |
| cottage | 2 tablespoons | 4 | 30 |
| cream | 2 tablespoons | 2 | 110 |
| Butter | 1 tablespoon | 6 | 100 |
| Cream | 2 tablespoons | 1 | 60 |
| Ice cream, vanilla | 1/2 cup | 3 | 145 |
| | | | |
| **Protein** | | | |
| Meat, lean | 1 ounce | 8 | 80 |
| Liver | 1 ounce | 8 | 65 |
| Bologna | 1 piece | 6 | 155 |
| Eggs | 1 egg, medium | 6 | 80 |
| Dried beans | 1/2 cup, cooked | 8 | 115 |
| Peanut butter | 2 tablespoons | 8 | 190 |
| Peanuts | 1/2 cup | 19 | 420 |
| | | | |
| **Fruit** | | | |
| Fresh, unsweetened | 1 medium | 1 | 50-100 |
| cooked, sweetened | 1/2 cup | 1 | 100 |
| | | | |
| **Vegetables** | | | |
| Green, leafy vegetable | 1/2 cup | 2 | 20 |
| Beets | 1/2 cup | 1 | 25 |
| Corn | 1/2 cup | 3 | 85 |
| Potatoes | 1 medium | 2 | 80 |
| Peas and lima beans | 1/2 cup | 5-6 | 60-90 |
| | | | |
| **Breads and Grains** | | | |
| Bread, whole-grain or enriched | 1 medium slice | 2 | 60 |
| Cereal, cooked, whole-grain or enriched | 1/2 cup | 2 | 60 |
| Cereal, ready-to-eat, whole-grain or enriched | 3/4 cup | 1-2 | 80 |
| Crackers, plain | 2 crackers(medium) | 1 | 35 |
| Cookies, plain | 2 small or 1 large | 1 | 120 |
| Cake, un-iced | 2x3x1-1/2" piece | 2 | 200 |
| Cake, layer, iced | 1/16 of 10" cake | 4 | 370 |
| Pie, fruit | 1/7 medium | 3 | 350 |
| Pie, custard type | 1/7 medium | 8 | 280 |

# 5.

# NAUSEA AND VOMITING DURING PREGNANCY

**1.** *What causes nausea and vomiting during pregnancy?*

Nausea and vomiting during pregnancy are often called *morning sickness*. There is an emotional element that may be involved. We also think certain hormones may be secreted during pregnancy that cause the discomfort. In addition to these causes, digestion in general is slowed. Food often takes many hours to digest. In the meantime, it sits there and produces a sensation of fullness and bloating. Sometimes your diet plays an important role. In some women, it makes little difference what they eat—nothing digests well.

**2.** *How long does morning sickness last?*

It may begin early in pregnancy and continue until your body adjusts to the vast amount of hormonal change. Ordinarily this takes about 12 weeks. Some fortunate women never experience nausea.

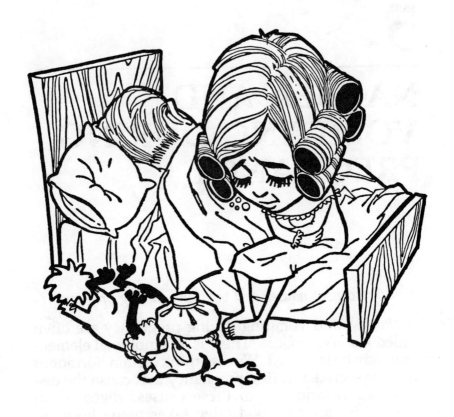

*Is morning sickness really in my head?*

### 3. Is morning sickness really in my head?

If it is, then over 60% of all pregnant women have something wrong with their heads. Although you might concede a certain emotional element, it is unfair to say all nausea is in a woman's mind. Such statements usually come from men or from women who have never experienced the feeling. Morning sickness is not limited to morning. Most women feel better as the day progresses.

### 4. If nausea is severe with one pregnancy, does it mean it will be severe with the next pregnancy?

Not always, but this is often the case. Sometimes a tense home situation, marital difficulties or unwanted pregnancy tend to make the nausea more severe.

### 5. When are nausea and vomiting dangerous?

If nausea and vomiting persist, they cause weight loss and a serious upset in the electrolyte balance in the body. The latter occurs because too much hydrochloric acid is lost from the stomach.

In some cases, hospitalization becomes necessary to overcome the imbalance. Intravenous fluids and sedation help correct the situation.

Unfortunately, it is not uncommon to find nausea and vomiting recur after leaving the hospital. Symptoms usually subside after 12 to 14 weeks of pregnancy.

### 6. What can I do about nausea during pregnancy?

It depends on how severe the nausea is. Some women have nausea when they get up in the morning. For them the answer is to get rid of the early morning stomach residue by vomiting. After this, they feel better and often have no further nausea or vomiting for the rest of the day.

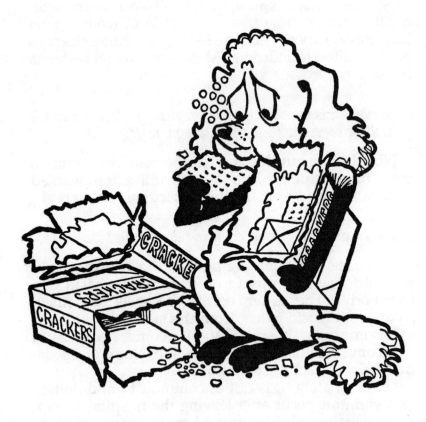

*What can I do about nausea during pregnancy?*

Other women find it helpful to avoid fried or greasy foods, as well as rich desserts. Still others are helped by eating small, frequent meals that keep something in the stomach. Crackers, Melba toast, Coke syrup or thick, cooked cereal are sometimes helpful. Most liquids taken while you are nauseated do not stay down.

If you find no relief with simple measures, a shot of vitamin B6, with or without vitamin B1, may help.

## 7. *What about severe cases of nausea?*

In extreme cases, it may be necessary to hospitalize the patient. There she will be fed intravenously and her electrolytes (her body chemicals) will be carefully balanced.

Only very rarely is abortion necessary in these cases. It is performed only for prolonged, persistent or resistive nausea and vomiting during pregnancy.

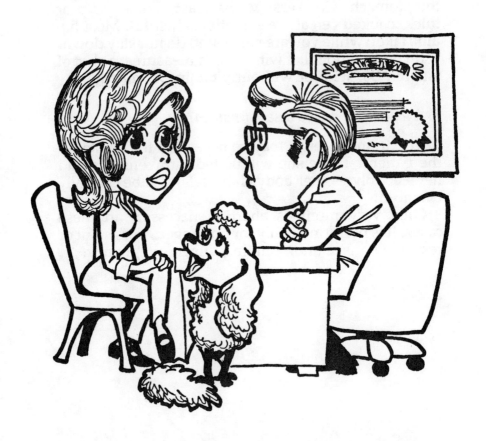

*Do most women take medicines during pregnancy?*

# 6.

# MEDICINES IN PREGNANCY

No unnecessary drugs should be given during pregnancy, but it is important that necessary drugs not be withheld from you or your fetus. If you understand about drugs and pregnancy, you will also understand why your doctor gives you certain medicines and advises against others during pregnancy.

1. *Do most women take medicines during pregnancy?*

One survey showed the average pregnant woman takes four or five different medicines during pregnancy. About four out of five drugs taken by women in pregnancy are taken on their own, rather than by a doctor's prescription.

2. *Do all the drugs I take pass to the fetus?*

As far as we know, most drugs pass through the placenta to the fetus in some amount. The placental barrier between you and baby is *not* a barrier to drugs.

3. *Drugs don't cause all defects, do they?*

No. For instance, certain diseases, such as German measles, cause defects. Heredity also plays a role in defects. X-rays, some industrial chemicals and other environmental factors can also cause defects.

4. *How early in a pregnancy can drugs pass through the placenta to the fetus?*

Drugs can pass freely either way through the placenta by the 5th week.

*Anytime* after conception the baby could be affected by drugs. Early in pregnancy, from conception to implantation in the lining of the cavity of the uterus, a drug can *kill* the embryo. After the 11th day, drugs are more likely to cause defects.

This can occur before you missed a menstrual period or are even aware you are pregnant.

5. *Are results of taking drugs predictable?*

Not always. Results depend on many factors, including:
- Type of drug.
- Dose of drug.
- Time of gestation (how far along in pregnancy).
- Resistance or sensitivity of the fetus to particular drugs.

6. *At what point in pregnancy is my baby most likely to be harmed by drugs?*

Usually during the first trimester—the first three months—the fetus is most susceptible to drugs.

7. *How do drugs cause defects in the fetus?*

We do not know for certain, but there are several theories. We know that drugs can cause harm by:
- Reducing the oxygen-carrying capacity of the blood.

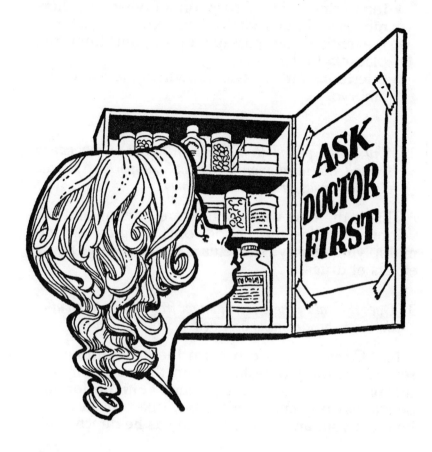

*What about aspirin, cold tablets, laxatives and other over-the-counter medicines?*

- Reducing the amount of sugar in the blood.
- Interfering with absorption of vitamins, hormones and other vital substances.
- Preventing the passage of oxygen from the placenta to the fetus.
- Interfering directly with growth of the cells of the embryo.

8. *Why is the period from the third week of pregnancy through the third month especially important for the fetus, as far as drugs are concerned?*

This is the time when organs are forming and developing. During this period, cells are growing and multiplying rapidly. The fetus is more sensitive to the effects of drugs.

9. *Does this mean there is no danger from drugs taken after the first three months of pregnancy?*

No. Certain drugs can harm the baby during the second and third trimesters—from the fourth through the ninth months of pregnancy. Your doctor understands drugs and their actions. Take *only* the drugs he gives you, and take them only as he directs you.

10. *Can it be predicted which organs of the baby will be affected according to the time in pregnancy when the drug was taken?*

Within certain limits, this is possible. The *nervous* system is most likely to be harmed from the 15th to the 25th week. The *visual* system, the eyes, is most likely to be harmed from the 24th to the 40th week. The *heart* is most likely to be harmed from the 20th to the 40th week. The *legs* are most likely to be harmed from the 24th to the 36th week.

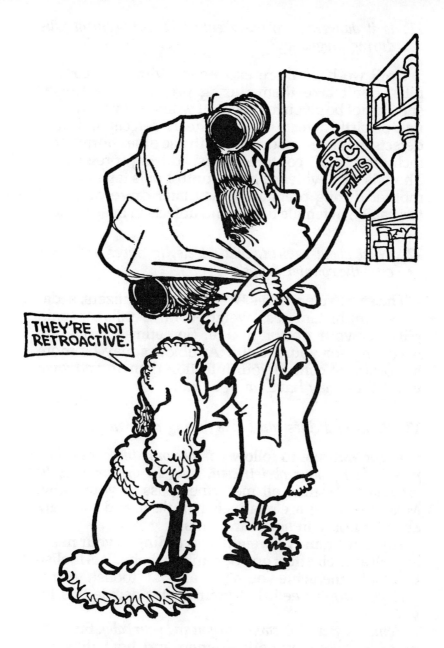

*Is it dangerous to mistakenly take birth-control pills during pregnancy?*

## 11. *Is it dangerous to mistakenly take birth-control pills during pregnancy?*

Until we have more experience with birth-control pills, don't take them during pregnancy. Estrogen should not be given to pregnant women. An increased risk of birth defects, such as heart defects and limb defects, has been associated with use of sex hormones, including oral contraceptives, during pregnancy. There is also evidence birth-control pills taken by the mother during pregnancy may later cause cancer of the vagina in female babies and defects in male babies.

## 12. *What about aspirin, cold tablets, laxatives and other over-the-counter drugs?*

The same rule applies. Whether tranquilizers, sedatives, antihistamines, weight-control pills or pain pills, let your doctor decide. Sometimes drugs are necessary for your health. Antibiotics may be more important to control your infection than any adverse effect they may have on your baby.

## 13. *What medicines can I take during pregnancy?*

A general rule to follow is: *Take only those medicines prescribed by your obstetrician, only in the amounts he prescribes.* Assume all medicines pass to your baby. Most medicines are relatively harmless, and some are absorbed only in small amounts.

All drugs must be weighed according to your need, as well as their effect on your unborn baby. It is foolish to avoid a medicine you need, and it is foolish to take one you don't need. Let your doctor decide this for you.

*Some drugs are life-saving to you and your baby.* But they must be taken properly—when and how they are prescribed by your doctor.

# 7.

# WHAT MAY I DO?

1. *Pregnancy is spoken of as a delicate condition. What am I supposed to avoid?*

Pregnancy is a normal physiological state. You can usually do anything during pregnancy you do when you are not pregnant. However, studies show blood may be directed away from the uterus to other muscles during strenuous exercise. Do not overdo it.

If you are used to tennis, golf, swimming or bowling, for example, these sports won't harm you or your pregnancy. It's better not to undertake new, strenuous activities that overtax you or your strength. Discontinue any activity when you are tired.

2. *What about bicycling, horseback riding and skiing? Are these too vigorous?*

If you are accustomed to them and in good physical condition, they won't hurt you during pregnancy. However, you should know whether these sports are difficult for you, even when you are not pregnant.

Usually people are thinking of miscarriage when they ask these questions. A normal woman carrying a normal pregnancy is not likely to miscarry, regardless of her activity. Women have tried most means to abort an unwanted pregnancy, usually without success.

If there is something wrong with a pregnancy, a woman will probably miscarry, whether she remains in bed or is active. All sports or activities should be discontinued when the bag of waters breaks or when contractions are five minutes apart.

3. *What about climbing stairs in pregnancy?*

Going up and down stairs is good exercise for the average, normal pregnant woman. If stairs prove too difficult for you, avoid them when possible. Sometimes a woman has excessive relaxation of her joints, which results in loss of some support and stability. If this occurs in your hips, you may find it difficult to walk.

Never look at the stairs when you are going up or down. Before you start, look them over, then look straight ahead. Keep your chin parallel to the stairs, then proceed up or down. Use the handrail.

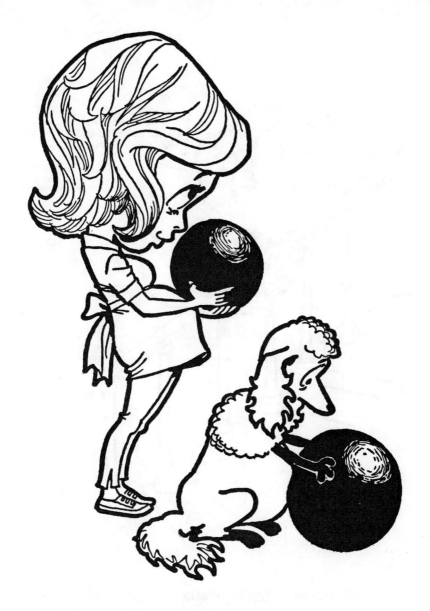

*Pregnancy is spoken of as a delicate condition. What am I supposed to avoid?*

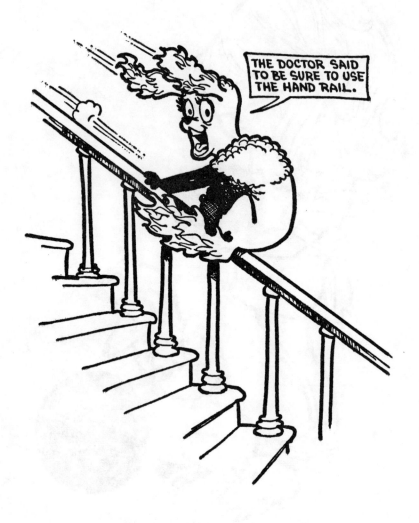

*What about climbing stairs in pregnancy?*

4. *What about swimming during pregnancy? Will it cause infection?*

Swimming is an excellent exercise for a pregnant woman. Because of buoyancy, swimming is less strenuous and more relaxing than many other sports. There is no evidence it causes infection—other than athlete's foot, if you are susceptible. Swimming is a good breast and chest exercise. Even the breast stroke, done out of the water, is beneficial.

5. *Can I continue to run while I'm pregnant?*

Running is all right if you are used to it. Walking is just as beneficial and more desirable, especially during the last half of your pregnancy.

6. *What exercises can I do during pregnancy?*

There are many different types of conditioning exercises you can do, from walking and swimming to a program of exercises designed especially for pregnant women. HPBooks publishes another pregnancy book, *Pregnant & Beautiful! How to Eat Right, Stay Fit & Look Great,* which deals with exercising and conditioning during and after pregnancy.

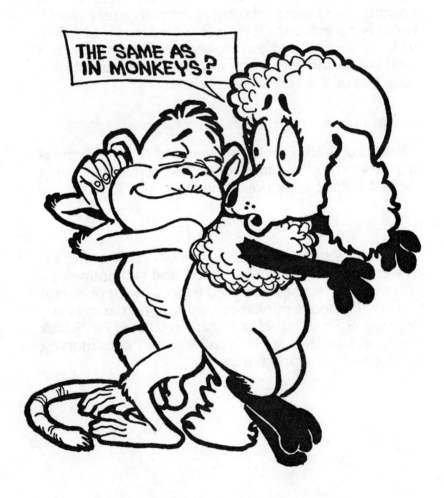

*Where did the name "Rh" come from?*

# 8.

# THE Rh FACTOR

### 1. *What does Rh mean?*

"Rh" is one of many substances called *factors* found in red-blood cells. The Rh factor covers a red-blood cell like a coat of paint covers a golf ball.

### 2. *How common is the Rh factor?*

There are several different Rh factors, and everyone has some of these. The most important one is called the *Rh D-factor*. About 85% of all human beings have this coating, which means 15% do not have it. Individuals who do not have this particular Rh factor are said to be *Rh negative*.

### 3. *Where did the name come from?*

It was named the Rh-factor because it was originally discovered in the blood of Rhesus monkeys.

## 4. Why is the Rh factor important?

The chemical coating of the red-blood cells produces an antibody response when introduced into the system of someone who does not have it. Antibodies are like reserve soldiers called out to protect the body against the intrusion of foreigners. In this case, the foreigners are the Rh-coated, Rh-positive, red-blood cells.

The body may tolerate a few foreigners. If many enter the bloodstream, usually by way of a leak in the afterbirth, an alarm is sounded. The body's reserve troops, antibodies, are quickly produced. This response becomes important in the following instances.

**Transfusions**—Blood containing the Rh-positive factor is not given to people who do not have it. The person receiving the Rh-positive blood transfusion would manufacture antibodies against the factor. This is called an *immune response*. The individual becomes sensitized against the Rh factor. If an Rh-positive blood transfusion is given to this Rh-sensitized person, anti-Rh antibodies would be produced by the body. The patient could suffer a severe, possibly fatal, reaction from this response.

**Pregnancy**—If an Rh-negative woman marries an Rh-positive man, they may have an Rh-positive child. Ordinarily, the blood of the fetus does not come in contact with blood of the mother. They have individual circulatory systems separated by a layer of tissue in the placenta.

A small leak could occur in the placenta, allowing some of the baby's blood to enter the mother's circulatory system. The two incompatible bloods would meet, and conflict could occur, similar to the above-mentioned transfusion. This can occur in the course of pregnancy, during labor and delivery or immediately after delivery.

The result is the mother, who does not have the Rh factor, treats the baby's blood, which *does* have the Rh factor, as a foreign element. This causes a reaction. The mother's Rh-negative blood responds to the baby's Rh-positive blood as though it were a vaccination. The mother's blood produces antibodies against the Rh factor coating of the baby's red-blood cells.

The antibody response is part of the body's vital defense system. It acts like a reserve army that quickly goes into action to protect its homeland from invasion by foreign agents. This is similar to the body's response to invasion by bacteria or viruses.

### 5. *Why is this antibody response dangerous to the baby?*

Antibodies are produced by the mother for her protection. The mother has no way of controlling their effect on the fetus, and the fetus is treated as an enemy of the mother.

Anti-Rh antibodies, produced by the mother, pass freely through the placental barrier between the blood of the mother and fetus. When these same anti-Rh antibodies reach the bloodstream of the fetus, they act like an army of retaliation. The result is they *destroy* the baby's Rh-positive, red-blood cells.

In an effort to compensate for this loss, the fetus speeds up the production line, turning out *incompletely formed* red-blood cells, called *erythroblasts*. From this process comes the name of the disease—*erythroblastosis fetalis*. It causes the fetus to produce incompletely developed red-blood cells.

This process may be compared to a production line in a factory that hastily turns out poorly assembled automobiles that never function the way they should.

### 6. *Is there anything to do to prevent Rh-sensitization in the mother?*

Yes. The mother can be given anti-Rh antibodies to combat the invading Rh-positive baby's red-blood cells. Then she will not have to manufacture her own antibodies. This is called *passive immunity*. This immunity is temporary, and the ready-made antibodies disappear after a few weeks. This is similar to giving a person tetanus antitoxin to prevent tetanus when he steps on a rusty nail.

If sensitization in the mother is prevented, she will not produce anti-Rh antibodies, which might destroy the red-blood cells of the next Rh-positive baby the mother might have. In other words, erythroblastosis is prevented before it can develop.

This is similar to importing mercenary soldiers to handle a temporary emergency. They are no longer needed when the emergency is over. After their job is done, they leave the country.

### 7. *Is there a shot that will give the mother passive immunity?*

Yes. Hyperimmune gamma globulin, also called *RhoGam*, can be given within 72 hours of birth of an Rh-positive infant to its Rh-negative mother. It is also given to unsensitized mothers at 28 weeks of pregnancy to provide immunity in the 5% of women who become sensitized late in pregnancy.

### 8. *Where do the antibodies come from that are found in RhoGam?*

These are human anti-Rh antibodies obtained from people who have developed an active immunity against the Rh-factor.

### 9. *How long does passive immunity last?*

Probably only for a few weeks, but this is the period during which sensitization occurs. If a non-sensitized Rh-negative mother has an injection of immune anti-Rh antibodies immediately after each Rh-positive baby, the next baby will be protected against erythroblastosis.

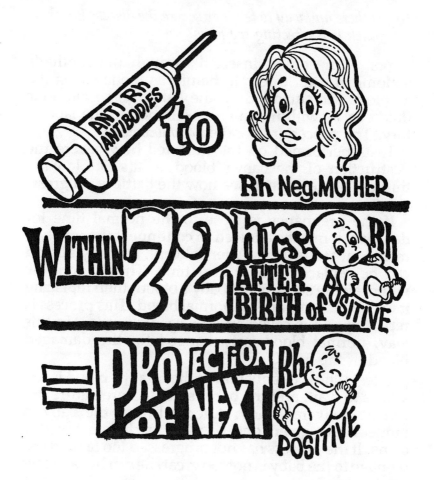

*Is there a shot that will give the mother passive immunity?*

10. *Is there any way to tell how severe the disease is or how much it is affecting the fetus?*

Yes. A needle is inserted through the mother's abdominal wall, through the uterus, penetrating the amniotic sac surrounding the baby. Some amniotic fluid can be withdrawn and examined in the laboratory. The procedure is called *amniocentesis.*

Tests performed on the fluid tell how severe the destruction of the baby's blood is. It's like looking through a telescope to see how the battle is progressing.

If the pregnancy is close to the normal time for delivery, it may be allowed to continue if the involvement is not too severe. After delivery, the baby's blood can be replaced a little at a time. This is done by withdrawing some of the baby's blood, then replacing it with equal amounts of normal blood. This process is repeated and is called an *exchange transfusion.* In this way, normal blood is exchanged for the damaged blood of the baby.

If tests show destruction of the infant's blood is too severe to wait, and the baby is not too premature, he can be delivered early. After delivery, the baby is immediately given one or more exchange transfusions. If the process has not progressed too far and the damage to the baby is not too great, he can be saved by the transfusions.

If the baby is too premature for delivery, he can be given a blood transfusion while still in the uterus. To accomplish this, a special needle is inserted through the mother's abdomen and uterus, into the baby's abdominal cavity where normal red-blood cells are deposited for absorption and use by the baby. Some babies require several transfusions to keep them alive until they are mature enough to survive at delivery.

To sum up what we know, Rh is a chemical coating found on the red-blood cells of 85% of all human beings. These individuals are Rh-positive. The remaining 15% are Rh-negative.

The Rh factor can provoke an immune reaction if it gets into the bloodstream of a person who does not have this factor. This is called *sensitization*. Sensitization becomes important in transfusions and pregnancy. It can result in severe reactions or even death of the mother or unborn baby.

The problem can be eliminated in transfusions by *never* giving Rh-positive blood to an Rh-negative individual.

Already sensitized pregnant women must be treated by early delivery of the baby in some cases. Intrauterine transfusions can be given to the fetus in severe cases in which the baby is too premature to be delivered.

Most non-sensitized Rh-negative mothers can be protected against sensitization by providing passive immunity against the Rh factor. This is done by giving them hyperimmune gamma globulin (RhoGam) within 72 hours after the birth of every Rh-positive child. This protects the next Rh-positive child against erythroblastosis.

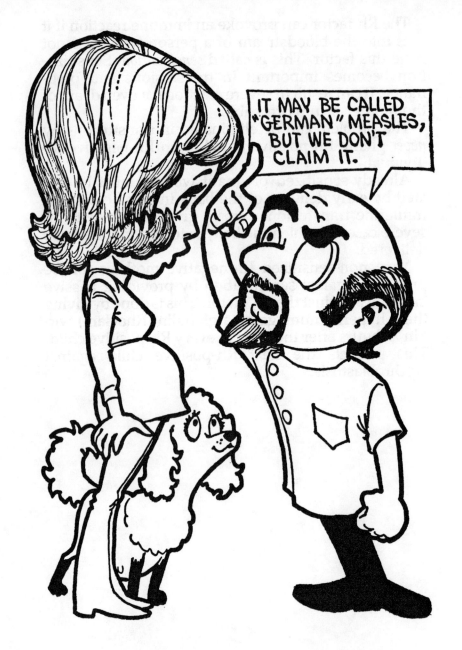

*Rubella is neither German nor measles!*

# 9.

# RUBELLA (GERMAN MEASLES) DURING PREGNANCY

German measles, also known as rubella, has been called "German" measles since the early 1800s. A German scientist pointed out the differences between this disease and regular measles, scarlet fever and a few other diseases. But it is neither German nor measles.

**1.** *What is the incubation period of rubella?*

Normally two to three weeks after exposure. The exposed person can spread the disease even if he shows no symptoms.

**2.** *What are some of the symptoms?*

All or none of these symptoms may occur—light rash, slightly raised temperature, some swelling of the neck, general discomfort, headache, sore throat, redness of the eyes and loss of appetite. If any of these symptoms appear, they last about three days.

### 3. *If I have rubella, how long can I infect others?*

Contagion is possible for at least two weeks after the rash appears or for four to six weeks after the original exposure. Some evidence indicates an infected person can continue to spread the disease for months.

### 4. *Would my doctor be able to tell if I have rubella?*

Diagnosis cannot be based on symptoms, which are often irregular, minimal or even non-existent. Accurate diagnosis is possible only by isolation of the virus from body tissues or by blood tests. In one epidemic, many infected infants were born to mothers who were totally unaware they had had rubella during pregnancy.

A new technique, the HI test, tests blood and detects immunity years after the infection. Your doctor can order this test.

### 5. *What is the treatment of rubella?*

Unless complications occur, rubella seldom requires any treatment beyond rest and recuperation. Complications are not as common as with measles, but they did appear with some frequency in a 1964 epidemic.

### 6. *Why is rubella so dangerous for pregnant women?*

Rubella produces few, if any, symptoms in the mother, and it may be passed to the fetus. It can cause death of the fetus or defects in a large percentage of babies.

In the rubella epidemic of 1964, it was estimated that about 20,000 babies were born in the United States with severe birth defects. An estimated 30,000 fetuses died. This was before rubella vaccine was available.

## 7. What defects does rubella cause?

**Hearing Loss**—Unless it is in the form of total deafness, as is often the case, the loss of hearing may not be discovered until the child reaches school age, when hearing is tested.

**Vision Loss**—This includes blindness, cataracts, glaucoma, abnormally small eyeball, retinal defects and corneal clouding.

**Heart Defects**—Sometimes heart defects are not apparent at birth. They are a frequent cause of death during early infancy.

**Abnormalities of Central Nervous System**—This includes brain damage that results in cerebral palsy or mental retardation. Another common deformity is abnormally small head size.

## 8. Will I know if I have rubella while I'm pregnant?

You probably won't. You may develop a mild pink rash and some fever, but there are many other diseases that produce these same symptoms. The only way to be certain is to have a blood test for the disease.

## 9. What should I do to protect future pregnancies against rubella?

There is a vaccine that will protect you against the development of rubella.

## 10. What about a rubella shot for me during pregnancy?

This should *never* be given during pregnancy. Even when you are not pregnant, you should not have a rubella shot unless you are willing to practice careful contraception for three months. There is a slight chance the weakened virus can get through to the fetus. The possibility of defects due to this is still under investigation.

Because 80 to 90% of women are already immune to rubella, every woman should have a test to determine immunity *before* she is given the vaccine. This will avoid unnecessary shots.

### 11. *What if I'm already pregnant?*

You should *not* be immunized. Although we think there is no danger of damage to your baby, it is best *not* to take chances. Pregnant women should not receive the vaccine.

### 12. *What if I'm not sure if I am pregnant?*

Do not take the vaccine. If it is given to an adult woman of child-bearing age, it should be given right after her menstrual period and only if she is willing to take birth-control precautions for at least three months.

### 13. *Should everyone be vaccinated?*

No. By age 11, about 80% of the population has had rubella and has a natural immunity against the disease. By age 20, about 92% of the population has been immunized in the same manner.

We must identify those who are not immune and have them immunized. This can be determined by a blood test. Those who are immune need no treatment or precautions. A blood test for rubella is part of routine prenatal care.

### 14. *What about immunization of children?*

Beginning at the age of 1 year—after natural immunity has worn off—and up to age 9 is the best time for immunization. After these ages are immunized, a continuous program of immunization of all 2-year-olds might eliminate the menace.

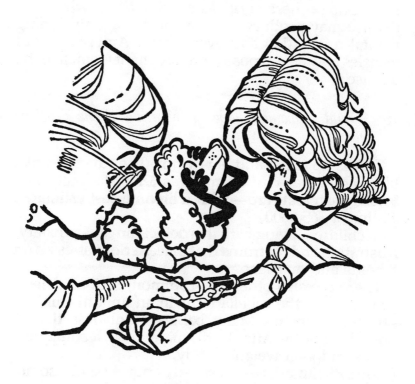

*Should everyone be vaccinated?*

15. *Are rubella parties, where children are exposed to German measles, safe?*

This is not recommended because there can be serious complications from rubella, though they are rare. One of these is *rubella encephalitis*, in which the disease may produce permanent damage, including mental retardation and even death. An epidemic of measles may also expose more pregnant women to the disease.

16. *Should a woman have an abortion if she develops rubella?*

This is up to her and her doctor. The education of a blind child may cost as much as $20,000 a year, plus $5,000 custodial care—with a lifetime cost estimated at almost $650,000.

In children, living with this defect can cause anxiety, frustration and tantrums that place serious stresses on a home and marriage.

There are also other less-common, serious defects produced by the rubella virus in an unborn child.

**Stunted Growth**—Many babies weigh less than 5 pounds at birth. After birth, many have feeding problems and gain weight slowly.

**Purple Birthmarks**—These red or purple spots, sometimes called *wine stains*, are often found on the face. They are caused by a bleeding tendency associated with low blood platelets, the blood's natural clotting agent.

# 10.

# HUSBANDS AND PREGNANCY

1. *When I'm trying to conceive, our lovemaking takes on a greater dimension. How can I make our relationship this ecstatic at other times?*

As your observation proves, emotions play a great role in sex. Perhaps this shows that you *can* enjoy sex on other occasions if you're willing to set the stage, put forth the effort and make it a truly fulfilling experience for both of you. It can be done!

2. *Will intercourse make me miscarry?*

Usually, no. If there is uterine bleeding or excessive uterine contractions following intercourse, your doctor may recommend you forego coitus. If a woman is threatening to miscarry, there is a possibility miscarriage could occur. If the pregnancy is normal, a woman will usually carry it to term. If the pregnancy is abnormal, she will usually lose it regardless of what she does.

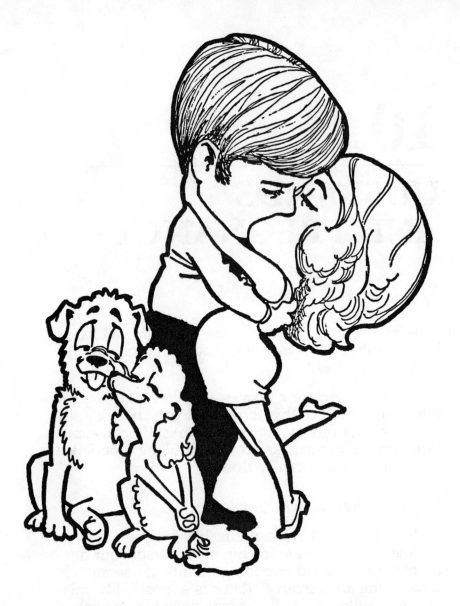

*My husband seems to love me more, now that I'm pregnant. But I'm afraid we might harm the baby. Are there any restrictions?*

3. *My husband seems to love me more, now that I'm pregnant. But I'm afraid we might harm the baby. Are there any restrictions?*

I assume you mean in lovemaking. No, there are no restrictions unless lovemaking is painful, but it should not be. If it is, check with your doctor to find out why.

Intercourse during pregnancy is normal and even beneficial for both of you. Frequently, you will feel closer at this time than at any other time during your marriage.

4. *Is it normal to dislike sex during pregnancy?*

No. This usually stems from a subconscious fear of harming the baby. This will not occur. If you can't overcome this fear, discuss it with your doctor. It is normal for some women to have a decreased libido during pregnancy.

Most couples enjoy sex more during pregnancy because the problem of birth control is eliminated. During most pregnancies, they feel closer to each other.

5. *Is there danger of infection from intercourse, especially toward the end of pregnancy?*

No. There is no evidence to show this occurs, unless the bag of waters has broken or there is some bleeding. Normally, you are more likely to have a discharge with itching during pregnancy. This does not seem to be due to intercourse, and it doesn't affect the baby.

Occasionally both husband and wife pass an infection back and forth, but this can be diagnosed and effectively treated during pregnancy. For more information on vaginal infections and vaginal discharge, see section *Vaginal Problems in Pregnancy*, beginning on page 99.

**6.** *Is it better to avoid intercourse during the first three months of pregnancy, while the baby is forming?*

No. This is a time when you should feel close to each other. Because we have no proof of harm done by intercourse during pregnancy, it is all right to continue it as though you were not pregnant. If you have any concerns, discuss them with your doctor.

**7.** *Should we stop having intercourse during the last six or eight weeks of pregnancy?*

Do you want to? There is no medical reason that you should. If it becomes too uncomfortable for you in the latter stages of pregnancy, use a little ingenuity. Try other positions and continue relations.

If you are especially protuberant, your husband may find he can enter your vagina from the rear, causing little or no discomfort to you. If he is gentle and you are not uncomfortable, sex should be enjoyed until the bag of waters breaks or contractions are five minutes apart.

**8.** *Can I still have an orgasm, even though I'm pregnant?*

Some women find their libido and satisfaction heightened during pregnancy. This may occur because they do not have to worry about becoming pregnant. But sometimes fatigue interferes, or occasionally a woman feels unattractive.

Sex can continue during pregnancy. A thoughtful husband will help his wife, by digital clitoral stimulation when necessary, to achieve orgasm while she is pregnant.

If you are prone to miscarriage or premature delivery, you may have to forego orgasm, but not intercourse, during the first three months or last two months of pregnancy. In some women, orgasm provokes painful uterine contractions that could lead to miscarriage or early labor.

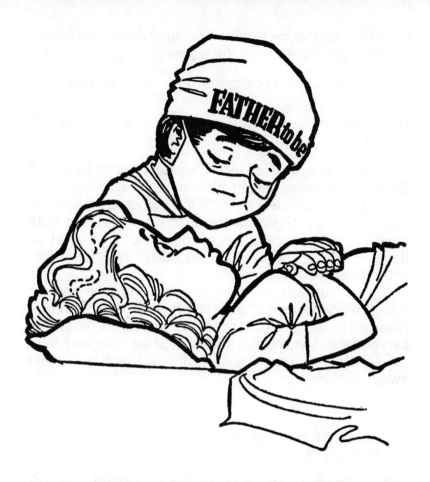

*Should my husband be allowed in the delivery room with me?*

**9.** *Is there any reason nipple stimulation during intercourse should be discontinued during pregnancy?*

No, unless this is distasteful to either of you.

**10.** *Should my husband be allowed in the delivery room with me?*

Do you want him there? Does he want to be there? Do hospital rules permit him to be there?

There are many advantages to having your husband participate and share this wonderful experience with you. However, some husbands do not wish to be there. Others, because of attitude and behavior, should not be there.

If your husband can be told what will take place in the delivery room and what role he will play, he can be comforting to you. Most men prefer standing or sitting by your side to give you support. Most women prefer to have their husband by their side, rather than farther away, looking on.

**11.** *Is there a book like this one for fathers-to-be that answers their questions?*

Yes. There is an excellent book available by Eric Trimmer, M.D. titled *Father-To-Be, Questions and Answers About Pregnancy, Birth and the New Baby,* also by HPBooks. The book answers many of the questions a potential father may have. It discusses his role in your pregnancy and the birth of your baby.

# 11.

# DANGER SIGNS OF PREGNANCY

1. *Are there any danger signs I should look for in pregnancy?*

Yes. Occasionally, a baby decides to complicate your life even before he is born. There are a few tricks a baby may try that cause symptoms your doctor will want to know about as soon as they occur. These symptoms do not necessarily spell problems. They indicate some treatment may be needed to *avoid* problems. Call your doctor if any of the following symptoms appear.

**Bloody Discharge from Vagina**—Early in pregnancy, this could mean a threatened miscarriage. Later, a bloody discharge could mean the afterbirth is in front of the baby, separation of the afterbirth before labor or the onset of labor.

In the first part of pregnancy, if bleeding is staining—less than the amount of your normal menstrual flow—the news can keep until morning. In the second half of pregnancy, notify the doctor immediately, regardless of the amount of bleeding. This does not include pink, mucoid discharge near the time the baby is due.

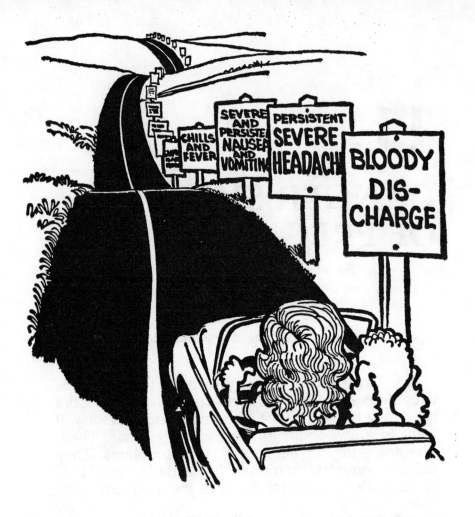

*Are there any danger signs I should look for in pregnancy?*

**Persistent, Severe Headache**—This can indicate toxemia of pregnancy, high blood pressure or, in rare cases, a brain tumor.

**Severe, Persistent Nausea and Vomiting**—This is discussed in the chapter on nausea and vomiting, beginning on page 51. When you vomit several times within a few hours, it is a danger sign. Report it immediately to your doctor.

**Chills and Fever Over 100F (40C)**—High fever can injure or even destroy a fetus. Report a high fever, particularly with a chill, immediately to your doctor.

**Swelling of Ankles, Feet, Hands and Face**—This can be an indication of toxemia of pregnancy and should be reported to your doctor. Puffiness of the face, eyes or fingers is significant if it is very sudden. Swelling of the legs and ankles when the face and hands are uninvolved *may* not be significant, especially in hot weather.

**Severe Abdominal Pain**—Unless it is a momentary catch or associated with constipation, report abdominal pain to your doctor. Pregnant women can have appendicitis and gall bladder attacks.

**Frequent, Burning Urination**—This usually indicates a bladder infection. Report it to your doctor to obtain effective relief from the symptoms. He will also prescribe a cure for the infection.

**Reduced Amount of Urine**—This can occur with or without increased thirst. If you are thirsty, your doctor will check for diabetes. If no diabetes is found, a decrease in the amount of urine can still be a serious sign. Let your doctor rule out any kidney trouble.

**Dimness or Blurring of Vision**—This is important in the second half of pregnancy.

**Sudden Gush of Water from Vagina**—This could indicate the opening of the membranes, resulting in the uncontrolled escape of watery fluid. When the bag of waters breaks, labor usually ensues, regardless of the duration of the pregnancy.

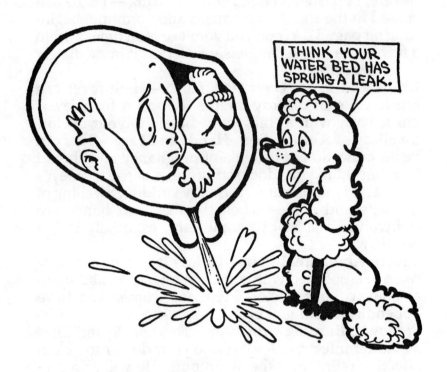

*Watch for a sudden gush of water from the vagina.*

## 2. *What are some rules to follow about calling my doctor?*

There are times when you *should* call him, and he would want you to. Below are a few suggestions.

- Except for emergencies, phone him at his office rather than his home.
- Give him your name and any other helpful information, the fact you are pregnant, how far along and when you were last in his office.
- If you cannot telephone the doctor yourself, have the person making the call well-informed about details. For instance, if the condition prompting the call is vaginal bleeding in pregnancy, you must let him know how much blood is being passed, if it is spots or streaks mixed with mucus, how it compares with the first day of a menstrual period and if there is pain associated with the bleeding.
- If your bag of waters has broken, tell him.
- If reporting uterine contractions, tell him how often, how long they last and how severe they are. Also tell him if you have any bearing-down sensations.
- If reporting about your urinary tract, tell him if you are passing blood, how much, how often you are urinating, how painful it is and if there is any pain in your back.
- Talk to the doctor yourself if possible. Relaying questions and answers back and forth through a third party may result in a misleading story for the doctor and garbled advice for you.
- Have a pencil and paper handy in case you must write down instructions.
- When calling the doctor, know the name, address and telephone number of your nearest pharmacy. Your doctor may wish to telephone a prescription for you. It will speed things up if you can promptly give him this information.

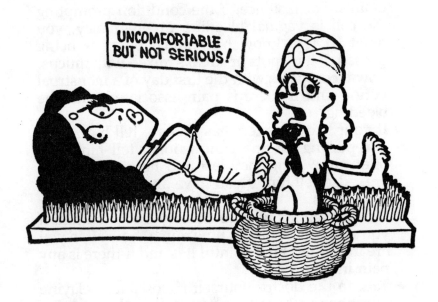

*Some symptoms of pregnancy are more uncomfortable than serious.*

# 12.

# SOME NORMAL DISCOMFORTS OF PREGNANCY

**1.** *Is it normal to be tired all the time?*

To some women, this is the first indication they may be pregnant. In many pregnant women, basal metabolism is slowed during the first three months of pregnancy. Your doctor will decide if you need thyroid medicine.

Don't worry if you require more sleep than you did before pregnancy. Try to take a nap during the day. Women who *never* get enough sleep can simply be happy they are not elephants. They have a twenty-two month gestation period for each pregnancy.

If fatigue is out of proportion, tell your doctor so he can check your blood and make any tests he thinks are necessary.

Sometimes, a small amount of fatigue is necessary to slow you down while you are pregnant.

## 2. Why doesn't my food digest?

Digestion is slowed, and often food feels as though it just sits like a lump in your stomach. Antacids may help, but check with your doctor first. Learn which foods agree with you and which foods do not, then eat accordingly. Eat small meals, eat more often and chew your food well. Avoid fried or greasy foods and rich pastries. Your digestion should return to normal after pregnancy.

## 3. Why do I cry so easily?

A pregnant woman's feelings are very fragile. You may cry easily, often and frequently without justifiable provocation. This calls for understanding on the part of your husband. Both of you must realize this is temporary and not serious.

## 4. I have never had constipation before. Why now?

Constipation is related to indigestion in pregnancy. The tone of the bowel muscles is diminished, and the bowel does not do its job as it should. Prune or orange juice and increased liquids may help.

Avoid harsh laxatives, as well as repeated enemas. Usually a bulk laxative that acts as a stool softener, such as Metamucil, will answer your needs. Be sure to check with your doctor before you take *any* medication or preparation.

## 5. Why do I have a backache all of a sudden?

The ligaments of your body do lose some of their tone and relax. As a result, they don't support your joints as they should. This is most noticeable in joints that bear weight, such as your pelvis and back.

Pregnant women often walk with their legs farther apart to compensate for the poor support and to retain their balance. They also have more pain in back and hips because of this lack of support.

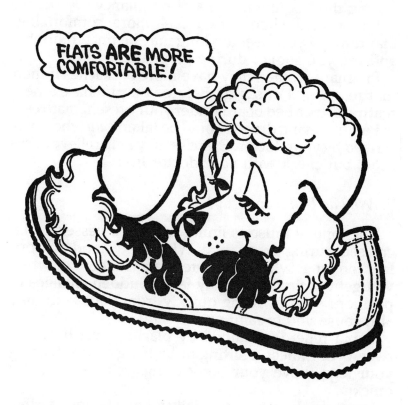

*Backache may be relieved by correcting your posture and wearing low-heeled shoes.*

## 6. What can I do for backache?

Correcting your posture often helps, but occasionally a brace or pelvic support is necessary, especially during the last few months of pregnancy.

Low-heeled shoes often feel more comfortable. Standing on your feet too long may be uncomfortable and tire you sooner during pregnancy.

Pregnant women may have more backaches if their mattress is soft or saggy. Before you purchase a new mattress, try a bed board under your present mattress.

Pain-relieving drugs should be taken *only* when prescribed by your doctor. Exercise may help relieve backache, but check with your doctor first.

## 7. Why do I faint so easily?

The tone of muscles lining the blood vessels is decreased during pregnancy. When you stand on your feet too long, when you enter a warm room or when you get too tired, you may faint. Sudden changes of position, such as rising quickly from your bed, may also cause you to faint or feel faint.

Rapid relief is obtained by placing your head between your knees if sitting or by lying down. Raising your legs above your body brings relief even more quickly.

Don't drink water, especially if you are only partially awake and alert. Never pour water into the mouth of a person who has fainted.

# 13.

# COMMON SEXUAL INFECTIONS AND DISEASES

There was a time when venereal disease meant either gonorrhea or syphilis, and that was that. The term venereal has been changed to *Sexually Transmitted Diseases (STD's)*, and the American Public Health Association now includes over 25 different diseases under this classification.

Let's begin with vaginal discharge in general, and then some of the more significant and common STD's of pregnancy. Many women will have a vaginal infection at some time during their pregnancy, regardless of personal cleanliness. Most of these infections can be easily diagnosed and controlled. Unpleasant symptoms can be quickly relieved. But in order to effectively treat a troublesome discharge, a diagnosis must be made.

1. *Is vaginal discharge normal, even when I am not pregnant?*

Yes. In a normal menstrual cycle, your body produces two hormones, estrogen and progesterone, both of which have an influence on your vaginal discharge. Before ovulation (when an egg is released), estrogen causes a colorless, watery discharge to be produced, a discharge that looks and feels much like raw egg-white. This discharge comes from the cervix and may become rather profuse.

By contrast, after ovulation this same discharge under the influence of progesterone, becomes white, opaque, sticky, and often less profuse in amount. During pregnancy this discharge can be clear or opaque and can vary in amount from scant to profuse, but is likely to be increased. Unless infected, however, it should not be irritating or cause itching.

As mentioned, such a symptomless discharge is normal and requires no treatment or special hygienic measures other than normal bathing and personal cleanliness. Douches and medication for a normal discharge are not always necessary and may even be harmful because they wash away the normal vaginal secretion.

2. *What is chlamydia?*

Unknown until just a few years ago, chlamydia has now become the most common vaginal infection. Public health officials estimate that 3 to 5 million Americans get chlamydial infections each year, making chlamydia far more common that gonorrhea, genital herpes and syphilis combined.

### 3. Why is chlamydia so important?

Due to chlamydial infections, 11,000 (some experts even place the figure at 35,000) women of childbearing age become involuntarily sterilized each year.

Due to chlamydial infections, 75,000 newborn babies per year will develop conjunctivitis (eye infection).

Due to chlamydial infections, 30,000 newborn babies per year will develop pneumonia.

Due to chlamydial infections, which also cause Pelvic Inflammatory Disease (PID), an infection of tubes, ovaries and surrounding structures, more than 200,000 women will be hospitalized this year and more than 1,000,000 will require treatment for PID.

### 4. How can I tell if I have chlamydia?

First of all you must realize that 60 to 80 percent of women with chlamydia have *NO* symptoms. The most-common symptoms are:
- Vaginal itching and discharge
- Painful and/or frequent urination
- Chronic abdominal pain (may be sign of pelvic inflammatory disease.)
- Bleeding between periods

Demand diagnostic tests if:
- You or your husband have what is called "acute urethral syndrome" (frequent, urgent, painful urination, along with a sterile urine specimen that contains pus).
- If you or your husband have gonorrhea (chlamydia often accompanies gonorrhea).
- If your husband has a "morning drip" type of penile discharge even if gonorrhea cannot be proved.

### 5. *How difficult is chlamydia to treat?*

Usually a 10-day treatment with erythromycin will cure the chlamydia. Remember that there is no immunity to chlamydia. It can recur and it can also lie dormant for years, then flare up when least expected. If your husband has chlamydia, insist that he wear a condom during intercourse until he is cured.

It is a good idea to have a follow-up smear, culture, or 30-minute Microtrak test after treatment, even though symptoms have disappeared, just to make sure the disease has responded to the treatment. Chlamydia can be cured!

### 6. *What about Trichomoniasis?*

Another common vaginal infection that can afflict all women, not just pregnant ones, is trichomoniasis. It is caused by a tiny turtle-shaped organism that can easily be seen when the discharge is examined under the microscope. Typical discharge is foamy, itchy and irritating, but responds readily to a drug called Flagyl.

Unless husband and wife take treatment at the same time, the infection will simply ping-pong back and forth and no cure will be obtained. However, Flagyl must not be administered to pregnant women during the first three months of their pregnancy. Partial relief at this time must be limited to simple douches and sanitary measures.

### 7. *Will trichomoniasis harm my pregnancy?*

There is some evidence that trichomoniasis may cause premature labor.

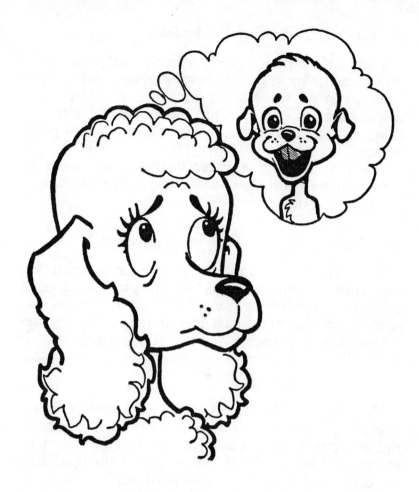

Tetracyclines, if taken while you're pregnant, may later cause discoloration of your child's teeth.

## 8. *What is Yeast Infection (Moniliasis)?*

Yeast infection is common in women, especially during pregnancy. It often occurs when penicillin has been given for some other infection. Yeast infection responds readily to nystatin, but treatment with this drug is best left until the last two trimesters of pregnancy.

The discharge in a yeast infection is similar in appearance to cottage cheese, and it causes itching, burning and discomfort.

## 9. *Will yeast infection harm my pregnancy?*

Yeast infection in a mother can be conveyed to her baby during birth and cause "thrush", which is a yeast infection of the baby's mouth and throat. There is also some evidence that yeast infection may cause premature labor, although this is still being studied.

## 10. *What is herpes infection?*

Herpes genitalis infection knows no age limit but is prevalent in pregnancy because women of childbearing age are more sexually active. Characterized by extremely tender, blister-like lesions on the lips, clitoris, cervix or thighs, herpes is also thought to be a risk factor in cancer of the cervix.

There is no cure for herpes, although acyclovir helps to control it. It may lie dormant for many months, only to flare up again when least expected. About 80 percent of victims of herpes have unpredictable recurrences, but each recurrence seems to be less severe until the disease just sort of burns itself out.

It is good to remember that herpes can be infectious even if the victim has no symptoms. It is estimated that about 5 million Americans have herpes.

## 11. *Will herpes harm my pregnancy?*

Herpes may cause abortion and increases the risk of cancer. If the herpes is transmitted to the fetus, it can cause death. For this reason cultures are taken from the 35th week on, at weekly intervals. If these cultures are negative, vaginal delivery may be undertaken, otherwise a cesarean section is performed in order to protect the baby.

## 12. *What about AIDS?*

AIDS stands for Acquired Immune Deficiency Syndrome, a condition in which a blood-born virus attacks and destroys the body's immune system. At the present time there is no cure. When the immune system has become sufficiently impaired, the victim dies from an "opportunistic" disease like pneumonia or cancer against which the individual normally would have good resistance.

Although we don't have a cure for AIDS, we do know a few things that will help to avoid catching it. For this reason, it is important to be as knowledgeable as possible about it.

There is a test that will demonstrate if you have been exposed to AIDS and whether you have developed "antibodies" against the disease. If you have been sexually intimate with anyone from a high-risk group (homosexual and bisexual men or intravenous drug users), you certainly should be tested.

If you test positive for antibodies, that does not mean that you have AIDS, only that you have been exposed to it. It takes from about 30 days up to six months after exposure to test positive for antibodies, so a negative test during this period of time might not be accurate.

The incubation period for sexually acquired AIDS is unknown, but it may range from 3 to 10 years, which means a long period of worry for those who test positive. Infants born to AIDS-infected mothers can develop the disease within the first six months of life.

Not all people who are exposed to the AIDS virus will develop antibodies to it, and not everyone with antibodies will develop AIDS, but indications are that about 20 to 30 percent will develop AIDS within five years. These figures could change as we learn more about the disease.

Since 1985 we have had accurate methods of checking for the presence of the AIDS virus and since that time, transfusions have been safe. If you and your husband have had a monogamous relationship for 10 years, you do not have to worry about the disease.

13. *Can AIDS be transmitted between couples during normal intercourse?*

Yes. About 7 percent of the cases have been traced to heterosexual transmission. It is easier for a man to transmit it to a woman than the other way around. If your husband tests positive for AIDS, it does not mean that he has the disease, but it does mean that he has been exposed to it and has developed antibodies against it. Insist that he use a condom during intercourse.

AIDS can be transmitted to your baby if you are pregnant and have the disease. Be sure to make your physician aware that you either have the disease or that you are at risk for it so that all precautions can be taken to prevent its spread.

# 14.

# MISCARRIAGE AND LABOR THAT STARTS TOO EARLY

A normal pregnancy is carried for 40 weeks or 280 days—counting from the first day of the last menstrual period until delivery. Normal variation is two weeks either way.

When the baby comes earlier than this, there is always some increase in risk of survival. In general, the earlier the baby comes, the less chance he has for survival.

1. *What is a miscarriage?*

Miscarriage is delivery of the baby before he weighs 1-1/4 pounds (460 grams) or before 20 weeks of gestation. This definition is more legal than medical because survival of the infant before 24 weeks is extremely rare.

2. *When is an infant considered to be premature?*

When he weighs between 1-1/4 pounds (460 grams) and 5-1/2 pounds (2500 grams).

3. *Why does a doctor often call a miscarriage an abortion, even though it happened by itself?*

Abortions are called *induced abortions* if they are intentionally performed. *Spontaneous abortions* occur by themselves. Whether spontaneous or induced, the correct medical term is *abortion*. The lay term is *miscarriage*.

Many people falsely interpret an induced abortion to mean a criminal abortion. Since abortion has been legalized, these are now called *therapeutic abortions*, which are abortions performed for the good of the mother or, in some cases, the baby.

Abortion carried out under favorable circumstances by qualified personnel is safe. Carried out under less-than-optimum conditions, abortion can lead to infection, chronic illness, sterility and occasionally death.

If abortion becomes necessary, seek competent advice. Have the procedure performed where facilities are well-staffed and well-equipped.

4. *What causes spontaneous abortions?*

Some common causes include abnormal egg, abnormal sperm or an abnormal union of the two. This is thought to account for 25% to 50% of all spontaneous abortions.

Abnormal conditions of the uterus and abnormalities in the afterbirth can also cause spontaneous abortions. In *placenta previa*, the fertilized egg is implanted too low in the uterus. This causes the afterbirth to lie ahead of the baby. If abortion does not occur, there may be severe hemorrhage in labor and delivery.

Early separation of the afterbirth before birth of the baby and clots in the blood vessels of the placenta are two other causes of spontaneous abortion. Abnormalities in the mother, such as infections, injury or an incompetent cervix, may make it impossible for the mother to contain a pregnancy within the uterus until the proper time for delivery.

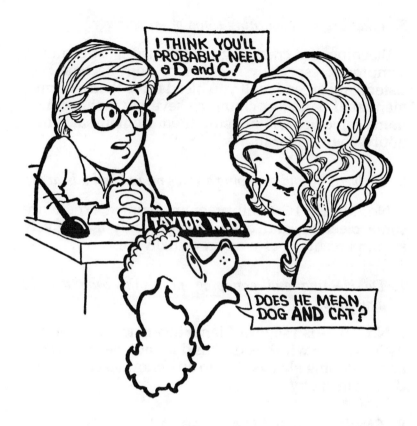

*What will my doctor do if I have a miscarriage?*

There are other causes, including hormonal imbalance, that we do not fully understand.

5. *What are some warning signs of miscarriage?*

Bleeding and cramping are the two most common symptoms, especially if either or both become persistent and excessive. If you bleed more than a normal menstrual period or cramp so severely that ordinary home-remedies will not stop them from intensifying, notify your doctor immediately!

6. *Do bleeding and cramping always mean I will miscarry?*

No. Nearly 1/3 of all pregnant women experience some bleeding and cramping, yet only a relatively small percentage of women actually miscarry,

7. *Do bleeding and cramping mean the baby will be abnormal?*

No. There is a slightly higher incidence of abnormality in women who bleed. This does not mean bleeding and cramping always lead to an abnormal child if you do not miscarry.

8. *Should I go to bed to avoid losing the baby?*

Let the doctor decide about this. Ordinarily, it makes little difference,

9. *Does it help to raise my feet and legs when I'm bleeding?*

No. This may only *conceal* bleeding by damming it in the vagina. It does not decrease the amount of bleeding or prevent miscarriage,

10. *What will my doctor do if I have a miscarriage?*

Usually, your doctor will take you to the hospital. There he can perform a D and C (dilatation and curettage) or a vacutage. These two procedures consist of stretching the cervix and removing the tissue involved with the pregnancy by scraping or with suction.

In most hospitals, early abortions are now performed by suction. This is often simpler and safer.

11. *Does a woman always have the uterus scraped after a miscarriage?*

No. Occasionally all the products of conception—the baby and afterbirth—are passed completely and bleeding stops. In this case, there is no need to scrape or suction out the contents of the uterus. Your doctor will decide whether or not this is necessary.

12. *How do I know I'm not going into labor too early?*

You may not know. If you begin having contractions that gradually become harder, closer together and last longer, you may suspect early labor.

13. *When is a miscarriage beyond hope for saving the baby?*

The pregnancy has probably passed the point of no return and will be sacrificed if placental tissue has passed, if bleeding becomes extremely heavy, if cramps become uncontrollable or if the doctor finds the cervix is already dilating.

14. *How do I know if the baby is too early to survive?*

This depends on his size, vigor and age. With improved methods of care for premature babies, more are being saved at earlier ages. Few survive if more than 12 weeks early.

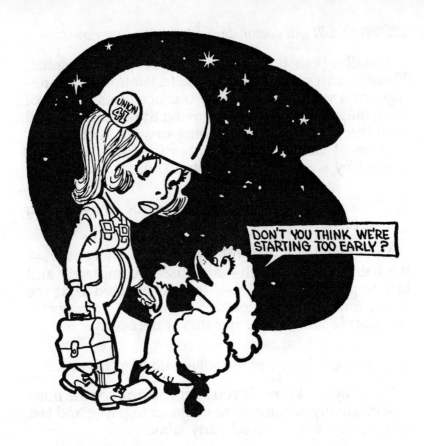

*How do I know I'm not going into labor too early?*

### 15. Does a "showing" always mean I will go into labor?

Not always. You may or may not lose the plug of mucus from the cervix. It often contains streaks of blood and is called a *showing*. Even though you pass the plug of mucus and have contractions, it is still possible you may not go into labor. Until the cervix starts to dilate, there is always a possibility of carrying your baby longer.

# 15.

# BLEEDING LATE IN PREGNANCY

Bleeding early in pregnancy, before the fetus is capable of survival, often indicates miscarriage. Bleeding in the last three months of pregnancy has a different meaning. In general, there are three types of bleeding late in pregnancy.

**The Showing**—With the onset of labor, a plug of mucus is dislodged from the cervix. It is often accompanied by streaks of blood, and is called the *showing*. Bleeding is slight and followed in a few hours by labor contractions. Your doctor will want to know if bleeding is present, even if it is slight in amount.

**Painless Bleeding**—When a woman has painless bleeding in the last three months of pregnancy, it may indicate the afterbirth or placenta lies ahead of the baby. This is called *placenta previa*. The condition could be serious and requires your doctor's immediate attention.

Tell your doctor how much you are bleeding, whether it is bright-red blood or dark, black blood and if it is accompanied by pain or not. He will determine if immediate delivery is necessary or if you may be allowed to wait and be watched.

**Bleeding With Severe Abdominal Pain—** Occasionally there is bleeding behind the afterbirth that causes it to separate from the uterus before the baby is born. This is called *premature separation* of the placenta. If enough of the placenta is separated from the uterine wall, it can no longer deliver enough oxygen to the baby, and the baby suffocates.

Along with pain, you may notice a stony hardness and extreme tenderness of the uterus. Notify your doctor at once if you experience this type of pain or bleeding.

### 1. *Are there other causes of bleeding late in pregnancy?*

Yes. There may be minor causes, such as erosion of the cervix, polyps (small berrylike growths) or varicose veins of the vagina that break and bleed. These can be taken care of by your doctor. Let *him* make the diagnosis and decide how important bleeding is. Also, when your doctor performs a pelvic examination during the last month of pregnancy, it may cause some bleeding for the next few hours.

### 2. *What do I tell my doctor about how much I am bleeding or how much blood I have lost?*

Report the amount of blood in terms of thoroughly or partially soaked pads, towels or underclothing. Or report the need for double padding or flooding through such padding every 15 minutes, half-hour or so. From this information, the doctor can judge whether it is an emergency or not.

If bleeding is more than light, he will probably want to examine you. In this event, take the soiled pads with you for examination, and let him evaluate the blood loss.

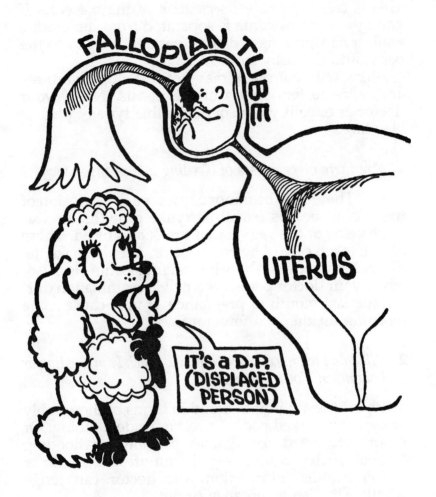

*Tubal pregnancy—the displaced person.*

# 16.

# TUBAL PREGNANCY— THE DISPLACED PERSON

A pregnancy anywhere besides where it should be, in the uterine cavity, is called an *ectopic pregnancy*. More than 90% of all ectopic pregnancies occur in the Fallopian tube. About one in every 200 pregnancies is misplaced.

## 1. *What causes tubal pregnancy?*

Apparently anything that delays passage of the fertilized egg down the tube to the uterine cavity can cause it to be implanted in the fallopian tube. Infection of the tube, an oversized egg and defective cilia (the small, hairlike structures lining the tubes that propel the egg on its way) are some common causes.

Some studies indicate tubal pregnancies are conceived late in the cycle. The ensuing menstrual backwash prevents normal descent of the fertilized egg through the tube into the uterine cavity, and an ectopic pregnancy results.

**2.** *What symptoms should I look for if I suspect a tubal pregnancy?*

One sign is a late, prolonged, different or even missed menstrual period. Another sign is pain on one side or the other, with or without bleeding. Before rupture of a tubal pregnancy, pain may be vague, mild or only a few cramps.

At the time of rupture, you may have what we call the *bathroom sign*. The sharp pain of rupture often occurs while straining with a bowel movement. Along with severe pain, you may faint or collapse on the floor due to the pain or sudden loss of blood when the pregnancy ruptures through the wall of the Fallopian tube.

When rupture of the tube occurs, it often tears through some blood vessels, which causes a rapid loss of blood. Nature drops the blood pressure, called *shock*, as a protective measure so you do not bleed to death.

This is an emergency and requires rapid diagnosis and treatment by transfusions and surgery.

**3.** *Why is a pregnancy test of little value in tubal pregnancy?*

A pregnancy test is positive only 35% to 40% of the time in tubal pregnancies. If negative, it does not mean there cannot be a tubal pregnancy. When the test is positive, it does not rule out a normal pregnancy in the uterus.

**4.** *Why does the doctor insert a needle into the vagina to make the diagnosis of tubal pregnancy?*

The needle is inserted through the wall of the vagina into the lowest part of the abdominal cavity to see if blood is present. Non-clotting blood obtained through the needle indicates hemorrhage in the abdominal cavity, which presumably comes from a ruptured tubal pregnancy.

5. *Does a tubal pregnancy always require surgery?*

Almost always. Rarely the pregnancy aborts into the abdominal cavity and bleeding stops. Ordinarily it distends the fallopian tube until it ruptures.

Bleeding usually continues until the blood vessels are *occluded*, which means until they are clamped or tied off at surgery. With rare exceptions, the diagnosis of tubal pregnancy requires surgery.

6. *If I have had one tubal pregnancy, am I more likely to have another one?*

Instead of one chance in 200, your chances of a second one are about one in 12.

7. *Is there any chance a tubal pregnancy can be carried to full term and a normal baby delivered?*

In the extremely rare cases in which this has occurred, the pregnancy became attached to the abdominal wall and continued to grow. However, such a pregnancy is hazardous because of the danger of hemorrhage even when delivered by Cesarean operation, as it would have to be.

When an ectopic pregnancy of any kind is diagnosed, surgery is done as soon as arrangements can be made. A blood transfusion may also be necessary.

8. *I've heard an intrauterine device (IUD) increases the chances of tubal pregnancy. Is this true?*

The incidence of tubal pregnancies was thought to be 10 times higher in women with an IUD, possibly due to infection. Recent statistics question whether the incidence is actually higher.

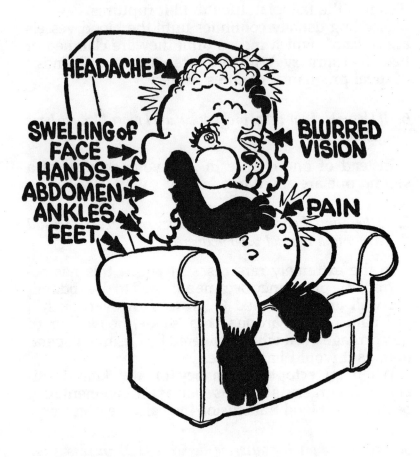

*How would I know if I had toxemia of pregnancy?*

# 17.

# WHAT IS TOXEMIA OF PREGNANCY?

Toxemia of pregnancy is a condition found only in pregnant women. Blood pressure is elevated, swelling and water retention occur and albumin appears in the urine. We do not know the cause, but we know how to treat it if we discover it early enough.

1. *How would I know if I had toxemia of pregnancy?*

Watch for swelling in your face, hands and abdomen. Headache is common, either in front or back. There may be a blurring of vision. Rarely temporary blindness occurs. Pain in the upper abdomen may occur. There will be a scanty amount of urine, even when you drink a normal amount of water. Report any or all of these symptoms to your doctor.

**2. Isn't some swelling normal for pregnancy?**

A small amount of swelling in feet and ankles is normal. Anything more than this should be reported to your doctor.

**3. What can I do to avoid toxemia of pregnancy?**

There is nothing we know of to avoid toxemia because we do not know the cause. If any of the three cardinal signs of toxemia appear—elevated blood pressure, albumin in the urine or swelling—you should report to your doctor immediately! Force fluids. Drink as much water as you can. Get adequate sleep and rest as much as possible.

**4. What if I don't improve, in spite of these precautions?**

Your doctor may have to put you in the hospital, where you can be observed and treated with medicine to control your blood pressure. If absolute bed rest and medicines do not control your toxemia, your baby may have to be delivered, either normally or by Cesarean operation, depending on your doctor's judgment.

**5. What happens if I ignore toxemia of pregnancy?**

If untreated, toxemia may become worse. Convulsions, coma and even death of the mother, as well as the baby, may occur. This is rare because most mothers are diagnosed early and adequate treatment is undertaken.

**6. Am I likely to have toxemia again with my next baby?**

About 1/3 of the women who have toxemia with one baby will have it with subsequent pregnancies. Women who have repeated toxemia of pregnancy are more likely to have a permanent elevation of blood pressure following pregnancy.

Toxemia of pregnancy is more common in women having their first pregnancy. Fortunately, these women have the least chance of having toxemia with subsequent pregnancies.

This does not mean every woman who has had toxemia with one baby will have it again. Nor does it mean a woman will have any aftereffects following toxemia of pregnancy.

7. *Is it possible to have high blood pressure and not have toxemia of pregnancy?*

Yes. These are two separate diseases, although they overlap somewhat. In the absence of disease, blood pressure has a tendency to become lower during pregnancy.

If you have high blood pressure, have a complete study of your condition before undertaking a pregnancy.

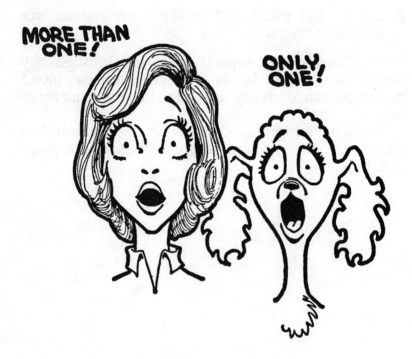

*More than one!*

# 18.

# MORE THAN ONE!

Generally speaking, the larger the animal and the longer it lives, the fewer offspring it has in its litter. Human beings are considered large and long-lived, hence our single-birth pattern.

1. *How can a doctor tell if I am going to have twins?*

He may be able to outline them through the abdominal wall with his hands. He may also be able to detect two heartbeats with his stethoscope. Electrocardiograms of the fetus' heart often detects twins. X-rays give *positive* evidence of twins. *Sonograms*—or ultrasound—are harmless and are often used in place of X-rays to diagnose a multiple pregnancy.

## 2. How common are multiple births?

Twins occur once in 99 deliveries in the white population and once in 74 in non-whites. They are most common in Blacks and least common in Asians. Triplets occur once in 10,000 deliveries, and quadruplets occur once in 1,000,000 deliveries. With the advent of fertility drugs, the incidence of multiple births is much higher.

## 3. What determines whether twins are identical?

When twins result from the splitting of a single fertilized egg, they are identical. Identical twins are always the same sex. However, when two separate eggs are fertilized, by two separate sperm, twins are fraternal—two brothers, two sisters or one of each. Fraternal twins are never identical.

Triplets, quadruplets or quintuplets may occur from various combinations of identical and fraternal twinning or from one, two or three eggs.

## 4. Which are more common, identical or fraternal twins?

About 25% of twins are identical, the other 75% are fraternal.

## 5. Are older women more likely to have twins?

Birth of fraternal twins increases in women between age 35 and 39, but decreases after the age of 40. Identical twins occur about the same percentage for all ages and races. The more children a woman has, the more likely she is to have fraternal twins.

## 6. How often does the doctor miss the diagnosis of twins?

Until the advent of ultrasound, about 50% of twins were not diagnosed until delivery. Now, the incidence of undiagnosed multiple pregnancies is much lower.

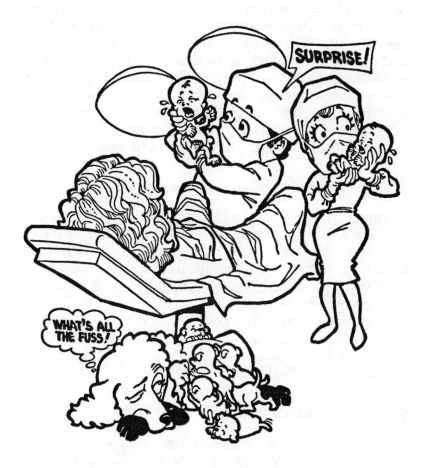

*How often does the doctor miss the diagnosis of twins?*

### 7. Will a twin pregnancy have more complications?

Yes. Twins are more likely to be born prematurely, so their chance of survival is a little less. Mothers of twins have a higher occurrence of toxemia of pregnancy, with its ensuing complications. Varicose veins and swelling—especially in legs—are more common in mothers with twin pregnancies. Defects are more common in identical twins. Twinning is considered a defect—but in this case, a desirable one. There is more false labor in twin pregnancies and more discomfort for the mother because of the large uterus.

### 8. Is there more hazard in delivering twins?

There is more likely to be compression of the umbilical cord due to entanglement. There are also more abnormal positions and more problems in delivery, such as prolapse of the umbilical cord, premature separation of the afterbirth with bleeding and a higher incidence of forceps deliveries.

Hemorrhage after twin deliveries is more frequent. Twin babies are smaller, usually because the mother goes into labor earlier. In general, twins have less chance for survival than a single baby.

### 9. Do twins share a placenta between them?

Each twin has its own placenta. The placentas may be located side by side so they look like one large, oversized placenta.

### 10. How can my doctor tell if twins are identical?

Usually this can be determined by microscopic examination of the membranes covering the babies. Fraternal twins have completely separate membranes. Identical twins share part of their membranes.

# 19.

# X-RAY AND ULTRASOUND

When X-rays are taken, an invisible beam of radiation passes through your body and is recorded on a film, like taking a picture. Shadows cast on this film outline bones and other structures. X-rays can be harmful to your unborn child if they are done in sufficient quantity and over a long period of time. Some X-rays may be necessary and even life-saving during pregnancy.

Ultrasound has replaced many former uses for X-rays in pregnancy, and it has been used for over 20 years to monitor the development of human fetuses. Ultrasound consists of high-frequency sound waves beamed into the pregnant uterus. The wave pattern is recorded as waves are bounced back by structures they encounter.

Experiments on animals using higher levels than pregnant women receive have shown some retarded fetal chromosomal growth, impaired immune response and chromosomal damage. Because of these results, Harvard obstetrician Dr. Fredric Frigoletto suggests, "Ultrasound should be performed *only* when definitely indicated, such as for diagnosis of suspected defects or to aid in amniocentesis."

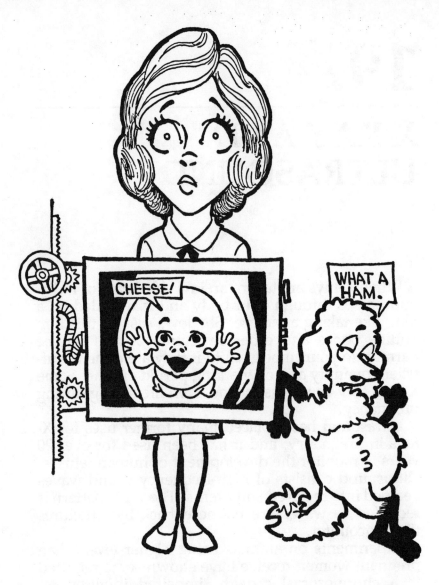

*Should I completely avoid X-rays during pregnancy?*

1. *Will X-rays hurt my unborn baby?*

The average X-ray, taken for diagnostic purposes, does not subject you or the fetus to a harmful dose. It is better to avoid all X-rays unless they are necessary, especially during pregnancy.

It would be foolish to neglect an X-ray when it is necessary to diagnose a condition that might require treatment. The radiologist will shield the pregnancy from X-ray exposure if possible.

2. *Are X-rays of my teeth or chest harmful to my baby?*

In general, irradiation reaching the pelvis from X-rays of the chest or teeth is much less than that received from water or air in the course of a week. But it is always wise to shield your abdomen when X-rays are taken, as a precaution.

3. *Are chest X-rays necessary during pregnancy?*

If there is a chance of tuberculosis, an X-ray of the chest may be needed for diagnosis. A newborn baby has no immunity against tuberculosis. To avoid exposure and possible death from the disease, it is worthwhile to take an X-ray of your chest, provided the abdomen is shielded.

4. *When is the best time to take X-rays in women?*

If possible, this should be done right after the menstrual period has started, before conception occurs. This is usually 14 days before the onset of the next expected menstrual period, and preferably no later than 10 days after the onset of a menstrual period.

5. *Should I completely avoid X-rays during pregnancy?*

Sometimes X-rays are necessary, such as in accidents, injuries, acute urinary tract infection or gall bladder conditions. Your doctor will weigh the benefits against the risk and decide if it is necessary during the pregnancy or if it can wait until after.

## 6. *Do X-rays later in pregnancy also cause damage?*

Most structures of the baby are well-formed after four months. Where possible, X-rays should be deferred until later in the pregnancy. Avoid unnecessary X-rays completely in pregnancy, regardless of the duration.

## 7. *Do X-rays cause cancer?*

Yes, but only in doses larger than those used in properly controlled X-ray studies. The use of X-rays is one of the greatest boons to health care in the past 50 years. Many of us owe our lives and health to X-rays. They are safe when used properly.

## 8. *What about ultrasound in pregnancy?*

Ultrasonography diagnosis is relatively new, but in the few years it has been used, it has proved a valuable diagnostic aid. Some research suggests ultrasound may affect chromosomes. This is still being investigated, but to date there is no evidence of damage to mother or fetus.

Ultrasound involves the same principles of sonar—sound navigation and ranging—used during World War II. High-frequency waves were beamed and bounced back by surface vessels to locate or track submarines.

In pregnancy, this "radar" is used the same way. It can measure the size of the unborn baby's head, diagnose early pregnancy, determine position of the fetus, diagnose twins, locate the placenta, diagnose death of a fetus, diagnose tubal pregnancy or detect certain abnormalities in the fetus.

Ultrasound is frequently used in place of X-ray and avoids exposure of irradiation. It is one of the valuable tools that enables your doctor to give you better care during pregnancy.

# 20.

# CESAREAN BIRTHS

*Cesarean birth* was once a frightening, dangerous experience. The procedure delivers the baby through an abdominal incision instead of the normal birth canal in the vagina. Today a Cesarean is one of the safest major operations. Even with the many serious conditions for which Cesarean may be performed, the mortality rate is only one in 400 operations. The incidence of Cesarean births may be as high as 15 to 20% in some places.

1. *Is it true once I have a Cesarean, I'll always have a Cesarean?*

If the same reason is still present, such as a pelvis that is too small, then the operation will have to be repeated with each pregnancy. If this indication is no longer present, it is the decision of your doctor whether or not to perform another Cesarean operation or to allow normal vaginal delivery.

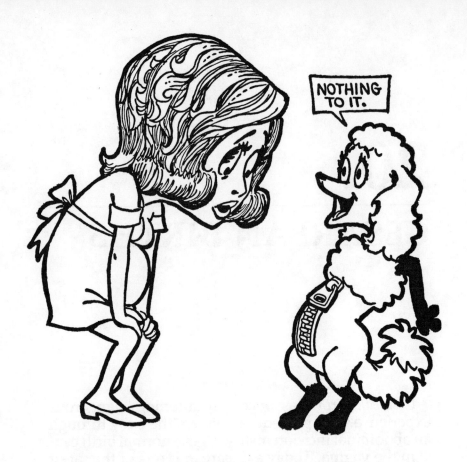

*Is it true once I have a Cesarean, I'll always have a Cesarean?*

**2.** *What is the most common cause of Cesarean delivery?*

A previous Cesarean birth. Depending on the method used for the first Cesarean operation, your doctor will decide whether to allow labor and vaginal delivery with subsequent pregnancies. Other causes of Cesarean may be a narrow pelvis, a large infant, unsatisfactory progress in labor, toxemia, placenta previa or prolapsed umbilical cord.

**3.** *Is there a greater risk to the baby with a Cesarean operation?*

This depends on the reason for the Cesarean. A higher fetal-mortality rate may not be caused by the Cesarean but may be due to prematurity of the infant, placenta previa with accompanying hemorrhage or many other causes. The Cesarean operation saves many infants who previously were lost in vaginal deliveries.

**4.** *How many babies can I have by Cesarean?*

There is no established limit. It depends on the condition of your uterus, how it has healed from past Cesareans, your general condition and other factors.

**5.** *Can a woman who has a Cesarean nurse her baby?*

Yes, and many do.

**6.** *Can a woman be sterilized when she has a Cesarean?*

Yes. The fallopian tubes are in perfect view and can be tied at the time of the surgery.

7. *Can the uterus be removed (hysterectomy performed) at the time a Cesarean is done?*

Yes. This is necessary in some cases. The operation carries a slightly higher risk than a Cesarean alone, but it is very successful.

8. *Is a Cesarean ever performed after death of the mother to save an infant?*

Yes. Failure to try to save the infant in event of death of a pregnant woman is considered negligence from medical and legal points of view.

# 21.

# WEIGHT AND SEE

A significant change has taken place in the medical profession's attitude toward diet and pregnancy. Only a few years ago, doctors placed great emphasis on limiting weight gain in pregnancy. This was done primarily to avoid toxemia of pregnancy. In the past few years, we have become more aware of the importance of adequate nutrition for the mother and fetus. Failure to meet nutritional needs of pregnancy may have far-reaching effects on an unborn child. Let's discuss this subject.

1. *Is excessive weight gain during pregnancy harmful to me or my baby?*

Yes. It is important not to gain too much weight. You may have a greater tendency to develop complications of pregnancy if you gain too much weight. It doesn't help your morale either to pile on unnecessary pounds of weight that are difficult to lose later.

There is a definite relationship between your weight gain and the weight of the baby. You could have a more difficult delivery because of the increased size of the baby.

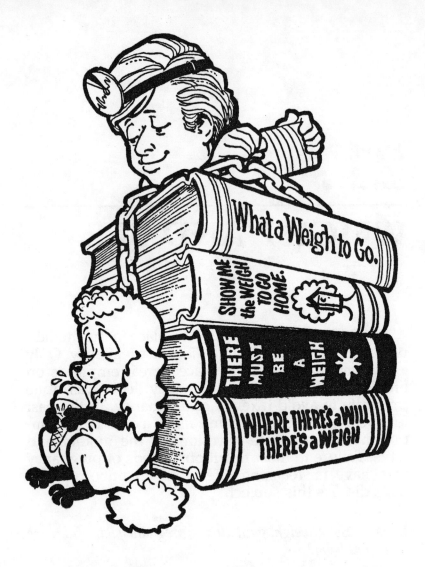

*What is considered an excessive weight gain?*

You may be asked to control your weight gain, but you will not be asked to lose weight. It is less risky for you and your unborn baby to gain extra weight than to diet and try to lose weight during pregnancy.

**2. *What is considered an excessive weight gain?***

It varies with each patient, depending on whether you are overweight to begin with, your general health, body build and stature, and other factors. Most doctors feel a gain of 24 pounds (10.8kg) for a pregnancy is normal. In general, a 24-pound weight gain in pregnancy is distributed as follows:
- Baby: 8 pounds (3.6kg)
- Placenta and membranes: 3 pounds (1.35kg)
- Amniotic fluid: 2-1/2 pounds (1.13kg)
- Uterus: 3-1/2 pounds (1.58kg)
- Blood: 4-1/2 pounds (2.03kg)
- Breasts: 2-1/2 pounds (1.13kg)

An average weight gain of 24 pounds is ideal. However, some overweight women may gain no weight, while an underweight woman may gain 30 pounds (13.5kg) or more. The optimum weight for you to gain will be determined by your doctor. Remember—never try to *lose* weight during your pregnancy!

**3. *Can I obtain sufficient vitamins from the foods I eat?***

You can and should. Because most processed foods are fortified with vitamins, this presents no problem. There are some cases in which your doctor may feel additional vitamins are needed.

**4. *What should I include in my diet?***

Try to eat protein for growth and repair of your body. Minerals and vitamins aid growth and keep your body in good working condition. Fats and carbohydrates provide energy.

---

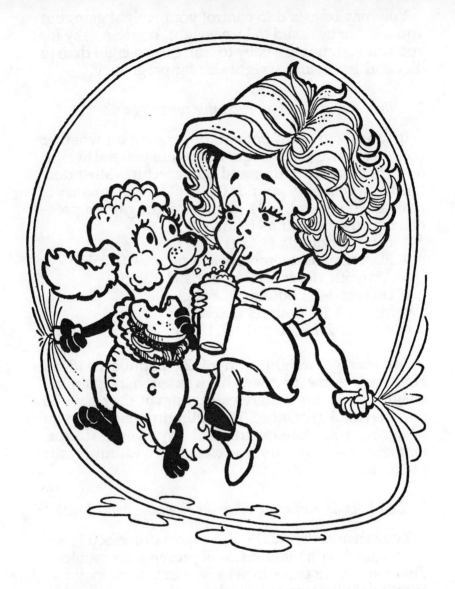

*Can you give me some hints to cut down on my caloric intake?*

A good diet contains a balance of these. Some women consult charts, but most pregnant women want a simple rule of thumb to direct them in preparation of healthy meals.

5. *What are the basic food groups?*

The basic food groups include the milk group, meat group, vegetable group, bread-and-cereal group, fat and oils, and sugars and sweets.

6. *Do some women need to pay special attention to their diet needs in pregnancy?*

Yes. These include:
- Women under 17 years of age who are still growing and maturing, in addition to meeting the needs of pregnancy.
- Women who have babies very close together. They may deplete normal reserves.
- Women who are underweight before starting a pregnancy. They have a double demand.
- Women who are overweight because their eating habits are faulty, and they eat too many sweets and carbohydrates. These women are often found to be protein-deficient.
- Limited-income women who may be trying to save money on food to meet other needs.
- Women who are anemic.

7. *Is it wrong for me to try to lose weight during pregnancy?*

Yes. There is usually too much danger of compromising the nutrition of the developing infant when you try to decrease your calories sufficiently to lose weight. This weight loss is better accomplished *after* the birth of your baby.

8. *Can you give me some hints to cut down on my caloric intake?*

Here a few suggestions that may help:
- Take an inventory of your eating habits.
- Choose a sensible diet pattern and include realistic exercise periods.
- Try changing your eating habits by shifting from three meals a day to five or six smaller meals a day.
- When possible, serve and eat meals buffet-style rather than family-style. This eliminates the temptation for second and third helpings.
- Use a smaller plate, and cut food into smaller pieces.
- Break the clean-plate habit. Leave a little food on your plate when you're finished.
- Make the meal last a long time. Most people eat less if they eat slowly.
- Drink water! It is assimilated quickly and aids digestion and elimination. It's also filling. Drink lots of water, especially when you get up in the morning and between meals. Water contains **no** calories!
- Never eat when you're overtired or upset. Try to relax before eating. Tension can undo many benefits of a well-balanced meal.
- Don't try to lose weight while you are pregnant!

9. *Are there any good books on nutrition during pregnancy?*

One of the best is *Pregnant & Beautiful! How to Eat Right, Stay Fit & Look Great,* also by HPBooks. It covers nutrition for the mother-to-be in detail and includes a section on post-partum nutritional needs for breast-feeding and bottle-feeding mothers.

# 22.

# HOW DO I KNOW WHEN TO GO AND WHAT TO DO?

There is one thing certain about pregnancy—it doesn't last forever. When you're pregnant, you know at some time you will start labor.

The big question with the first pregnancy is "Doctor, how will I know when I am really in labor?" It's a little like being in love. If you have to ask someone if you are, then you probably are not.

1. *How will I know when I'm in labor?*

True labor often begins with an intermittent backache or a feeling of discomfort in your abdomen similar to menstrual cramps. As your uterus contracts, your abdomen becomes stony hard. As the contraction ends, your abdomen feels soft again.

True labor contractions may be spaced at regular intervals, 8 to 20 minutes apart, and last over 30 seconds. It is important to time contractions both as to the interval between them and their duration. One reason they are called *labor contractions* and not *labor pains* is because they are not always painful.

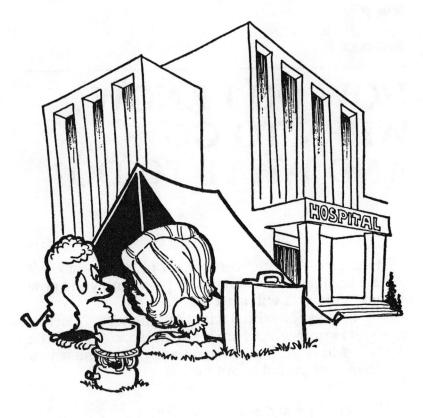

*How will I know when I'm in labor?*

If you feel intermittent backache or a tightening of your abdomen, place your hands over your abdomen and start timing. From the time the abdomen becomes stony hard until the time it again becomes soft is the *duration*. From the time the abdomen becomes soft until the time it becomes hard again is the *interval* between contractions.

Don't guess at the timing! You *must* be able to give accurate information to your doctor when you call him. When your contractions become regular at 5- to 8-minute intervals and last from 20 to 30 seconds, leave for the hospital.

Take into consideration how far you live from the hospital, how long it takes to get there and how uncomfortable you are. If you aren't able to relax between contractions, go to the hospital, regardless of whether contractions are regular or not! It might be a good idea to make a test run to the hospital to determine the best route and the driving time.

### 2. *Will I know when my baby drops?*

Several weeks before the onset of labor, the baby may drop or settle downward. You may or may not be aware of this. This change is the result of the baby's head descending into the pelvic cavity as the baby drops into a more favorable position for birth.

### 3. *Will I feel better or worse with this change?*

Upper abdominal pressure is often relieved when this occurs, causing your breathing to be easier. But you may also experience a more-frequent desire to urinate because of increased pressure on your bladder. You may also have cramplike pains in your thighs, and walking could be more difficult.

### 4. *What are Braxton-Hicks contractions and false labor?*

During pregnancy, it is normal for the muscles of the uterus to tighten intermittently. The uterus becomes almost stony hard, then relaxes and becomes soft again. This tightening is known as *Braxton-Hicks contractions*. Because they are mild, you may hardly notice them.

As the estimated date of birth approaches, these contractions may become cramplike and uncomfortable. Braxton-Hicks contractions are sometimes confused with true labor. Actually, it is just one of Nature's ways of preparing for true labor.

For a varying period before true labor is established, you may experience, and may be confused by, *false labor*. Unlike true labor, false labor pains usually occur at irregular intervals. They are confined mainly to the lower part of the abdomen and groin.

The duration of false labor contractions is usually short—30 seconds or less. Unlike true labor contractions, they are rarely intensified by walking and may be relieved by moving about or resting.

Instead of increasing in intensity, duration and frequency, false labor contractions diminish, then disappear completely. There may be several episodes of false labor over many days before true labor actually starts. False labor is less common in first pregnancies.

### 5. *What does the doctor mean when he says I'm dilated?*

"Dilated" refers to the cervix or neck of the uterus. As the uterus becomes tense and contracted, the force is referred to the cervix, which causes it to thin out, stretch and gradually open. The amount of opening is referred to as *dilatation*.

As the cervix dilates to allow the presenting part of the baby to pass through, it is measured in centimeters or inches. Full dilatation (cervix wide open) is a diameter of approximately 10 centimeters or 4 to 5 inches. This opening permits the baby to be born.

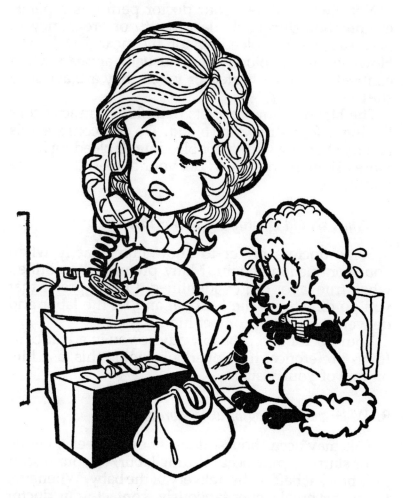

*When should I notify my doctor that I'm in labor?*

## 6. *Does a bloody show always mean I am in labor?*

Not always. When your doctor performs a pelvic examination during the last month of pregnancy, it may cause some bleeding for the next few hours. However, a true bloody show usually appears when contractions have started or when they are about to start.

The bloody show consists of a plug of mucus containing a few streaks of blood. Do not confuse this bloody showing with *active* bleeding. If bleeding looks more like menstrual flow, call your doctor. It could be important.

## 7. *When should I notify my doctor that I'm in labor?*

Some doctors prefer to know immediately when your contractions begin. Many prefer to be notified when true labor can be identified. Others prefer that you go directly to the hospital and let the labor and delivery personnel contact him.

Your doctor will probably advise you in advance as to his preference. If he overlooks doing this, ask him on one of your visits.

## 8. *When will my bag of waters break?*

This may occur hours, days, or even weeks, before labor starts. It may occur during labor, or your doctor may break it before the delivery of the baby. Whenever the water breaks spontaneously, contact your doctor or go to the hospital.

If you are close to term when your water breaks, your labor will probably start within 24 hours. If you are not at term, your doctor will decide the best course for you to follow. He will probably give you precautions to prevent infection if he allows you to go home to continue your pregnancy.

## 9. *What are different stages of labor?*

Labor is the process where the baby and afterbirth are expelled from your body. There are three stages of labor.

**First Stage**—The first stage begins when your cervix starts to open up or dilate. It ends when your cervix is fully opened or dilated.

**Second Stage**—This stage begins when your cervix is fully dilated and ends when your baby is delivered.

**Third Stage**—The third stage begins as soon as your baby is delivered and ends when your afterbirth is delivered.

## 10. *How long does labor last?*

The length of labor varies according to the size and position of the baby in relation to the size of your pelvis, how strong contractions are and how many babies you have had. Usually, each succeeding labor becomes easier.

Averages do not mean much, but beyond 24 hours for the first stage is considered abnormally long. Less than 3 hours labor is unusually short.

## 11. *What can I do to help my labor?*

Relaxation helps labor progress. Some women can relax during labor, others cannot. Many women are relaxed when they arrive at the hospital and check into the labor unit. In fact, some become so relaxed they wonder if their labor has subsided.

Because labor contractions are involuntary, they are more effective if not interfered with. Fear makes them less effective, and anxiety may prolong labor.

During the first part of your labor, relax as much as possible. Take deep breaths as contractions occur, and rest between them. To help accomplish this, try to unwrinkle your forehead, and allow your facial muscles to sag. This often helps relax other parts of your body. You may find it helpful to exhale a little more than you inhale.

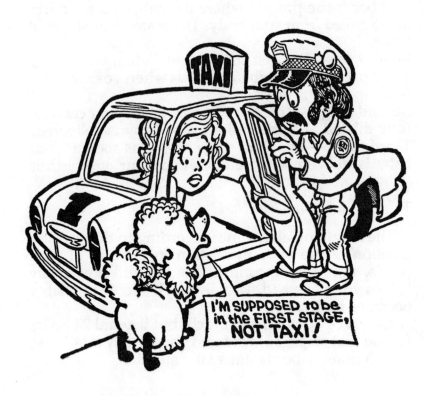

*What are different stages of labor?*

If you tighten your hands, you are less likely to relax. Place your hands over your abdomen or allow them to hang loosely at your side. Contrary to common belief, try not to grip your husband's hand.

## 12. *What about anesthesia for delivery?*

There is increasing interest in Lamaze methods and natural deliveries. In some cases, spinal and pudendal-block anesthesia cause a fall in blood pressure in the mother. This fall in blood pressure may also place the baby at risk.

Demerol, Nisentil and other drugs are used for relief of discomfort and often provide sufficient relief for delivery.

Epidural block, which means outside or on top of the dura (the covering of the spinal cord), is rapidly becoming the most popular method of anesthesia for delivery. Some hospitals have a full-time anesthesiologist on call to administer an epidural when needed.

Each obstetrician has been trained in his own particular method. Discuss anesthesia with him before your delivery.

## 13. *Will drugs to relieve pain harm my baby?*

If drugs are taken only as your doctor recommends, they are safe. However, do not insist on more medicine than you need. Often pain relief is requested when you are anxious and upset, rather than in pain.

A certain amount of almost every drug passes through the placenta to your baby. Although your doctor wants to relieve your discomfort, you want to ensure the safe delivery of your baby.

## 14. *Does it help to push with labor contractions?*

Not in the first stage. When your cervix is not fully dilated, pushing may stretch your bladder, rectum and pelvic floor, without helping to dilate your cervix. Pushing before you are told to may cause these organs to sag and lose their support after pregnancy.

## 15. *Will I be able to eat during labor?*

Food does not digest well during labor and tends to lie uncomfortably in the stomach. It is best to take only small amounts of clear liquids or a few ice chips.

If there is a possibility you will be having a general anesthetic, your doctor will probably ask you not to take anything by mouth after you start labor.

## 16. *What are birthing rooms?*

Birthing rooms are designed to include the family in a less-formal situation for delivery. Initially, these rooms were set up for women who wanted to deliver without a doctor, without anesthesia and without the availability of pain-relieving drugs.

Originally, many birthing rooms were used by licensed midwives. Today midwives still use them but many birthing rooms are also staffed by doctors.

Like other innovations, birthing rooms have changed and improved. Statistics show many women who wanted the advantages of a birthing room were forced to use regular hospital facilities because of various complications.

Recently there has been a trend by hospitals to accommodate women who prefer the informality of a birthing room with admission of their family for the delivery, along with Lamaze, drugless or other types of delivery. In these cases, the hospital birthing room combines the good points of each method. Doctors are in attendance or standing by, and anesthesia and analgesia are also available.

Transfusion, X-ray, laboratory facilities and other advantages of the hospital are available without losing the warmth of the birthing room. The birthing room has become one segment of a complete delivery division of the hospital.

17. *How safe is it to deliver at home?*

Home deliveries are a step backward. Although some reports statistically show home deliveries are safe, they give a false picture. Reports fail to take into account that complicated cases go to a hospital. Unplanned complications can and do occur, and often these complications require hospital facilities.

18. *Why is monitoring during labor and delivery important?*

Electronic monitoring has become a valuable part of every delivery division in modern obstetric care. There are two types of monitoring—*external monitoring* and *internal monitoring*.

**External Monitoring**—This is similar to a continuous fetal electrocardiogram. It provides a running report on the condition of the fetus and is accomplished by placing electrodes on your abdomen.

**Internal Monitoring**—This is accomplished with a tiny metal coil inserted into the baby's scalp through the mother's cervix. Internal monitoring is used when your abdominal wall is too thick, or it may be used in any situation in which an adequate record cannot be obtained through external monitoring.

A continuous monitor provides a constant record of the fetal pulse, contractions of the uterus and the response of the fetus to the pressure of contractions. It alerts your doctor when anything causes undue stress on the fetus, so stress can be relieved. This can mean anything from changing your position to performing an emergency Cesarean operation.

Monitoring acts as a watchdog for some otherwise undetected problems during labor and delivery. Monitoring has been responsible for saving the lives of many babies.

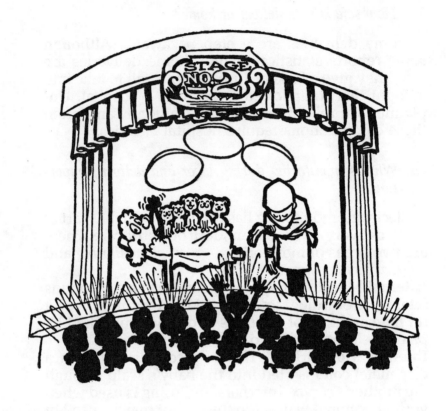

*Delivery—so this is how it is!*

# 23.

# DELIVERY— SO THIS IS HOW IT IS!

Delivery of the baby is another name for the *second stage* of labor. It is the actual birth of your baby through the vagina and consists of some twisting, turning, molding and expelling of your baby.

**1.** *How does my baby actually come out?*

Your baby usually delivers head first, with its crown making the first appearance. Next comes the forehead, with the brow, eyes, nose, mouth and chin appearing in succession. The baby "looks" down at the floor. See illustrations on following two pages.

The head then rotates to either side, and shoulders appear one at a time and are delivered. The rest of the baby's body follows the shoulders without difficulty.

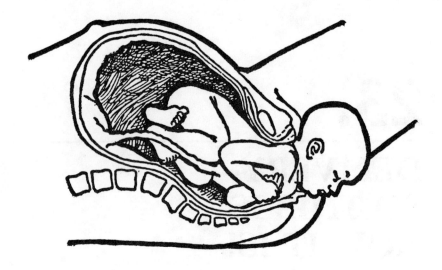

*Baby's head emerges first.*

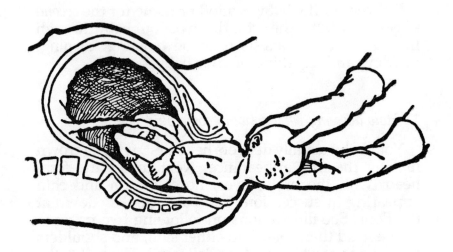

*Baby's shoulders deliver one at a time.*

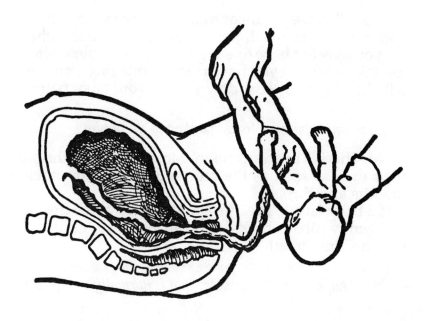

*Baby's body follows shoulders without difficulty.*

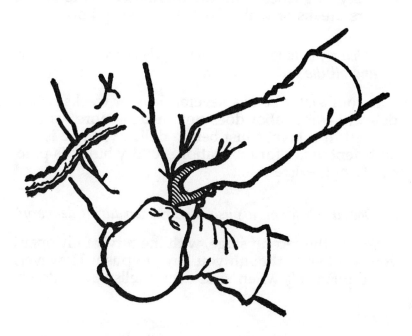

*Doctor carefully suctions mucus from baby's nose.*

**2.** *How do I know when my cervix is fully dilated?*

You will have an uncontrollable urge to bear down and expel your baby. If you have had a spinal anesthetic, you may not have this urge. However, your doctor can tell you when you have reached this stage, and he will direct you to "bear down" with your labor pains.

**3.** *Does my baby have to be spanked to make him breathe?*

No. This is a misconception. Most babies breathe on their own as soon as the mucus is wiped from their mouths and throats.

If a baby fails to breathe spontaneously, the doctor will gently rub his back—this causes him to gasp and take his first breath.

**4.** *What happens to all the water that is normally around the baby?*

If it has not slowly leaked out during labor and delivery, it gushes from the uterus when the bag of waters breaks or while the baby is being born.

**5.** *What is the danger of a dry birth if the bag of waters breaks and all the water leaks out?*

If your water breaks several days or weeks before delivery—and labor does not ensue—more water is formed. If it breaks just before delivery, there is still sufficient water for lubrication. A "dry birth" is practically non-existent.

**6.** *Does it help for me to push or bear down during delivery?*

Yes. In the second stage, with the cervix fully open, you will feel as though you have to push. However, try to push *only* when your doctor tells you to do so.

## 7. Should I massage my uterus to help it contract?

No. If such a maneuver is necessary, your doctor will take care of it.

## 8. What is an episiotomy?

An *episiotomy* is a cut made by the doctor from the opening of your vagina to the rectum to allow the baby to pass through more easily. If this cut is not made, the tissues must stretch to accommodate the baby's head. If tissue is unable to stretch sufficiently, it may tear into the rectum.

This procedure saves considerable pushing and straining on your part. It may also save injury to your baby due to prolonged pressure of the baby's head against rigid tissues.

An episiotomy wound is easy for the doctor to repair, and it will heal better than a jagged tear. The extent of an episiotomy is more easily controlled and thus prevents a tear into your rectum.

## 9. Is it better to let Nature take care of the problem? A woman is made to have babies. Can't I stretch that much without tearing?

Possibly. But then again, you might *not* stretch without tearing. It is also possible for your tissues to be overstretched so they do not return to normal. This leaves the supporting structures loose and saggy in the floor of your pelvis.

Sometimes the skin does not appear torn, but deeper tissues are torn, and they fail to heal together as they should. This also leaves a poorly supported pelvic floor. When this occurs, you may later have difficulty with your bladder and rectum or just a distressing feeling of "things falling out." An episiotomy prevents these complications and allows your doctor to tighten tissues that may have been overstretched or torn by previous deliveries.

A well-supported vagina and pelvic floor are also more desirable for satisfactory intercourse.

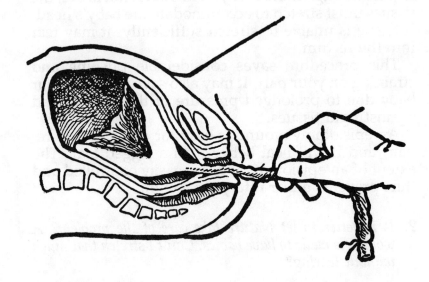

*After the baby is born, the placenta must be delivered.*

# 24.

# AFTERBIRTH— YOU MEAN THERE'S MORE?

Unless it has already been explained to you, you may be surprised to find you are not through with the "production," even though your baby has been delivered. There is still the matter of the placenta, or afterbirth, which must be delivered.

Usually the afterbirth is delivered spontaneously within 20 minutes after delivery of your baby. Rarely is it accompanied by more than a few cramps and moderate bleeding. Delivery of the placenta is called the *third stage* of labor.

1. *When is bleeding after delivery considered abnormal?*

Loss of more than a pint of blood is considered excessive, whether it appears rapidly or slowly over the next 24 hours. Sometimes a little blood covers a large area and appears to be a hemorrhage when it is not.

**2.** *Is there anything I should look for during the third stage of labor?*

Your doctor and nurse will watch you carefully. If there is a question in your mind or if you think you are bleeding too much, be sure to call their attention to it.

**3.** *What causes bleeding after the baby is born?*

**Atony**—One common cause of bleeding after delivery is failure of the uterus to contract and shut off open blood vessels. This is called *atony* or loss of tone in the muscular walls of the uterus. If the uterus remains boggy, the blood vessels that supplied blood to the afterbirth during pregnancy remain open and continue to pour out blood.

Massaging the uterus, along with certain drugs that make the uterus contract, soon stops this type of bleeding.

**Tears or Lacerations**—Another cause of bleeding is found in small or large tears that escape attention. These may be in the uterus, cervix or vagina. Examination by your doctor soon uncovers such bleeding, and a few well-placed stitches bring it rapidly under control.

**Retained Pieces of Afterbirth**—Another cause of bleeding is incomplete delivery of the placenta. If part of the afterbirth is left in the uterus, bleeding usually continues until it is removed.

Immediately after delivery of the placenta, the doctor examines it to make certain no pieces are missing. This is similar to examining a pie to make sure no piece has been cut from it. If the doctor determines part of the placenta is not there, or if he suspects there might be placental tissue remaining in the uterus, he will examine the uterus with his gloved hand and remove the fragment. Only in rare instances is it necessary to use an instrument to remove the tissue.

Occasionally, bleeding occurs when you are taken back to your room or even after you have gone home from the hospital. Report any bleeding that you think is excessive to your doctor or nurse immediately.

4. *Is there anything I can do to prevent hemorrhage?*

No. Sometimes a very rapid or very difficult labor will cause the uterus to fail to contract. A very large baby, a small pelvis, tissues that do not "give" or a very rapid delivery will sometimes cause tears. But your doctor can exercise skill in avoiding such tears, even when instruments are necessary. However, sometimes such complications are unavoidable.

Rarely there are clotting defects in your blood, and these must be corrected by your doctor. Your doctor has ways of testing for these defects and can usually correct them without difficulty.

In general, the best thing you can do is to cooperate fully with your nurses and doctor. They will do all they can to make your delivery as comfortable, safe and satisfying as possible.

5. *Will it help stop the bleeding if I raise my feet or raise the foot of my bed?*

No. It might conceal the bleeding for awhile, but it allows the blood to accumulate in your vagina. The blood may then come out in a gush when you stand up or go to the bathroom.

# 25.

# ABOUT NURSING . . .

**1.** *Will nursing make me lose my figure?*

This is a misconception. Support, or loss of support, and size of breasts is more often due to heredity and weight loss or gain. In general, there is no proof nursing will cause you to lose the contour, size or consistency of your breasts more than if you did not nurse.

**2.** *Is there anything I should do to prepare to nurse my baby?*

The most common problem is not the lack of breast milk but soreness of the nipples. Sometimes nipples can be toughened by soaking them in concentrated saltwater, but this may make them more irritated in some women.

Rubbing nipples with a dry washcloth or towel each day helps toughen them. Some women use Tincture of Benzoin with good results. Avoid lotions and ointments because they seem to soften nipples, rather than toughen them.

Massage breasts daily, especially if there is fluid—called *colostrum*—coming from the nipples. Try the exercises described below and illustrated on pages 166 to 168.

**Breast Massage**—Gently massage the breast to withdraw secretions from the nipple.

- Beginning above the breast, massage toward the **areola,** the pigmented area surrounding the nipple.
- Repeat massage, beginning underneath the breast. Lift breast as you massage it.
- Use both hands on sides of breast to massage toward areola.
- Repeat these exercises 10 times morning and night.

**Nipple Rolling Exercise**—This exercise will help improve nipple erectibility and keep milk ducts open.

- Use thumb and forefinger in rolling motion on nipple. Repeat 10 times morning and night.
- When finished rolling motion, use thumb and forefinger to withdraw colostrum.

3. *How should I take care of my nipples while I'm nursing?*

Washing before and after nursing is adequate. Do not use alcohol or harsh detergents. You can use mild soap, but be sure to rinse nipple thoroughly before letting the baby nurse.

If nipples become sore, use Tincture of Benzoin or an anesthetic ointment. By nursing on one side only, there will be more time for the sore nipple to heal. Allow the nipple to be exposed to the air by wearing a loose-fitting gown. A heat-lamp treatment may also help, but check with your doctor first.

4. *How long can I nurse my baby?*

It depends on how soon your pediatrician feels other foods can be added. Food is added as early as one month, in some cases. As early as four months, you may be able to start your baby drinking from a cup. This will eliminate bottle-feeding entirely, except for water in the earlier months. If you have an adequate supply of breast milk, you can nurse as long as you want. Many nursing mothers breast-feed their babies for the first year.

### 5. Can I nurse if I have very small breasts?

The size of your breasts usually has little to do with your ability to nurse. If you want to nurse, try it.

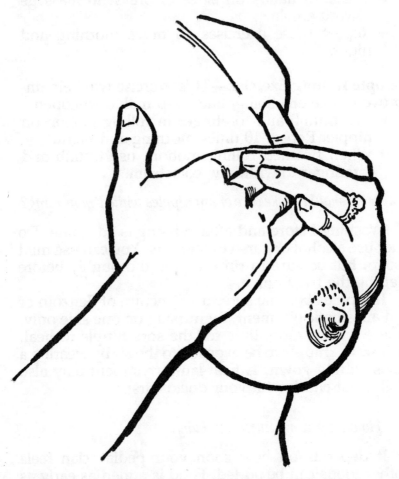

*Begin above breast, and massage toward areola (pigmented area surrounding nipple).*

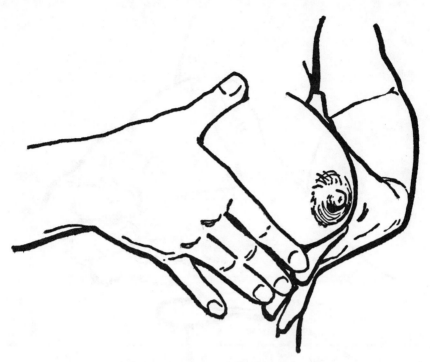

*Begin underneath breast, and lift breast as you massage.*

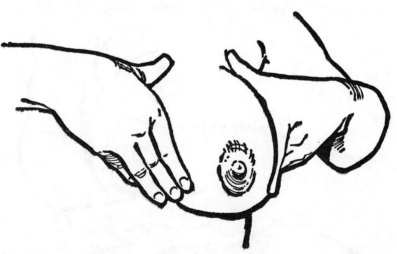

*Using both hands on sides of breasts, massage toward areola.*

*Repeat exercises 10 times morning and night.*

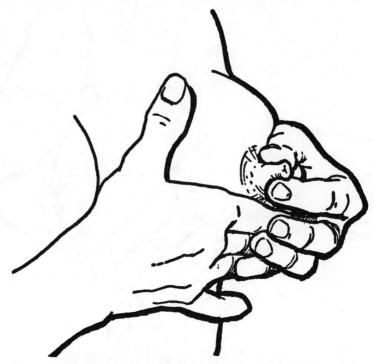

*Use thumb and forefinger in rolling motion on nipple to improve erectibility. Repeat 10 times morning and night.*

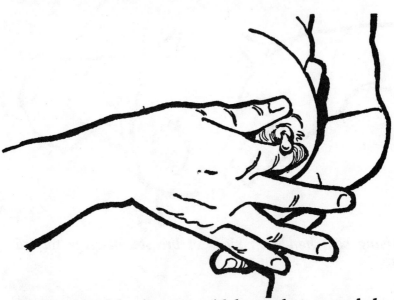

*Use thumb and forefinger to withdraw colostrum each day to keep milk ducts open.*

6. *How will I know if my baby is getting enough to eat when I nurse?*

In most cases, the baby will let you know. If he isn't getting enough breast milk, he'll be fussy and cranky. Otherwise, the scales will certainly tell the story.

7. *What if I don't have enough milk for my baby?*

The amount of breast milk will usually change to meet the demands of your baby. However, if your milk supply does not satisfy the baby, he will also do well on formula.

Although breast-feeding is desirable, it is better to have a happy, satisfied baby and a calm, relaxed mother than to struggle to nurse your baby on an inadequate milk supply or with breast milk that does not agree with him.

8. *Can I nurse twins?*

Yes. In most cases, your milk supply will increase to meet the demand of two babies.

9. *If I nurse, can I be away from my baby for a few hours or days?*

Yes. You may pump the milk and freeze it for the baby while you are away, or use formula. While you are away, pump your breasts several times a day to help you stay comfortable and to maintain your milk supply.

Traveling with a breast-fed baby may be easier than with a baby on formula. Your baby can become very portable when you breast-feed him.

10. *Will I get fat if I nurse my baby?*

No—unless you eat too much. It is not necessary to "eat for two" when nursing. A regular diet with plenty of liquids, even water, will usually produce sufficient milk for your baby.

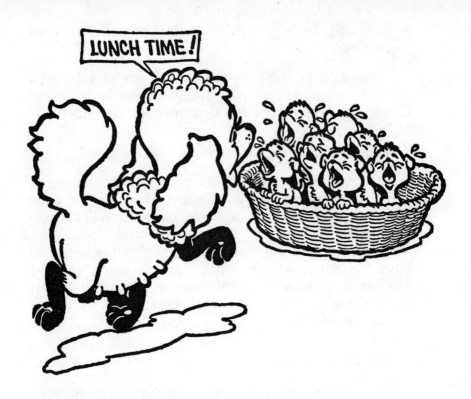

*How will I know if my baby is getting enough to eat when I nurse?*

11. *Must I be careful about what I eat if I nurse my baby?*

Most medicines are carried into your breast milk. Nicotine from smoking, alcohol and also laxatives find their way into your milk. These should be avoided, or at least minimized. Avoid chocolate and spicy foods, too.

12. *Are there advantages to breast-feeding?*

There are many advantages to breast-feeding your baby. It establishes a closer, more intimate relationship between you. Nursing also helps your uterus return to normal size and function faster. Bleeding is often less, and the decrease in the size of the uterus, called *involution,* is more complete in nursing mothers.

You need to take time out to sit down or lie down long enough to nurse your baby. There is some evidence to suggest mothers who nurse their babies have a lower incidence of cancer of the breast.

Many allergies are avoided when a mother nurses her baby. Sensitivity to certain milk products by the baby is also avoided.

Your breast milk is the one thing no one else can give your baby.

13. *Does breast-feeding save money?*

You could save a lot of money which you would ordinarily spend on formula and bottles if you breast-feed. You might be able to save enough money to buy a major household appliance or hire household help during the period you are nursing.

14. *Will nursing drain me of my energy?*

No. Many people think it does, but all new mothers get tired whether they are nursing their babies or not.

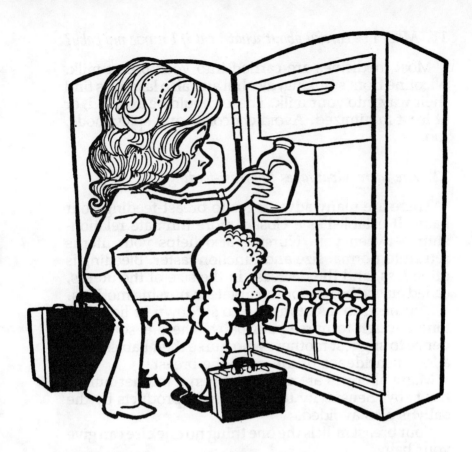

*If I nurse, can I be away from my baby for a few hours or days?*

Possibly a mother who must make formula, sterilize bottles and warm the milk gets a little more tired than the mother who cuddles her baby to her breast while she nurses him. There may be exceptions to this rule, however.

### 15. *If I nurse, will I be less likely to develop cancer?*

This is debatable. Some medical studies have suggested a lower incidence of cancer of the breast among nursing mothers. At least breast-feeding does not increase the risk of breast cancer.

### 16 *Can I nurse my baby even if I'm nervous?*

Yes. Tension may cut down on your milk supply and may prevent the milk from "coming in." It is important to learn to relax and get comfortable before nursing your baby.

Most women find breast-feeding calms them. It forces a busy mother to take time out from other responsibilities. You can cuddle, love and enjoy your baby while you nurse him.

### 17. *Is there any way to prevent sagging breasts after pregnancy?*

This is most often due to a hereditary lack of support. However, much of this sagging can be overcome by correct posture and wearing the proper bra.

A well-fitting bra is one that has broad, non-slip straps (padded, if necessary) over the shoulders and a broad, belt-type support underneath the cup.

Before your final selection of a bra, make sure straps stay in place and cups cover the entire breast when you raise your arms. If you nurse, buy a nursing bra to wear during pregnancy, which will allow for the increasing size of your breasts.

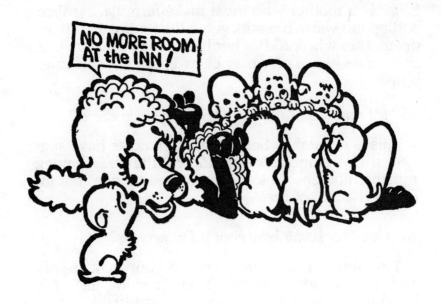

*Are there advantages to breast-feeding?*

18. *If I have a Cesarean, can I still nurse my baby?*

Yes. You may get off to a slower start, but there is no reason why you can't nurse if you want to.

19. *Will I be able to nurse, even though I have had silicone enlargement of my breasts?*

These envelopes are inserted underneath the breast tissue and should not interfere with nursing.

20. *How do I start to nurse my baby?*

A nurse will show you how to hold the baby and place the nipple in his mouth. Fortunately he already has a sucking reflex that tells him what to do from this point.

It's good to place the baby at the breast before the milk comes in, but be sure you don't allow him to suck more than a minute or his chewing reflex will make the nipple sore. Nothing seems to inhibit the supply of milk faster than sore nipples.

Allow the baby to get a good hold on the nipple, including the dark area (the areola). Otherwise, he won't be able to get much milk, and he will only irritate the nipple. When you want to discontinue nursing, break the suction by pressing some of the breast away from his mouth. To avoid pain to you, do not forcibly pull him away from your nipple.

21. *If my baby is premature, can I nurse him?*

Yes. Your breast milk can be expressed and sent to the hospital after it is withdrawn. When your baby comes home, he will quickly learn to nurse at your breast.

22. *Must I stop nursing when my baby begins teething?*

Not usually. Most babies don't usually think about biting the breast that feeds them. Others must be

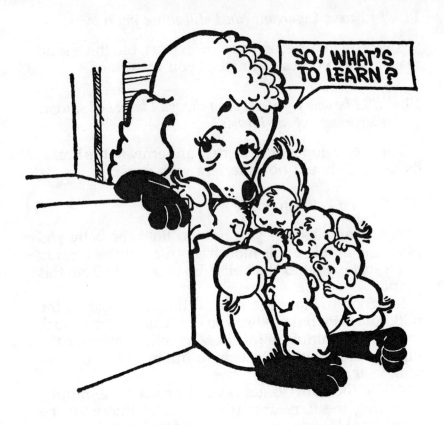

*How do I start to nurse my baby?*

taught—by taking them off the breast immediately, with an emphatic "No!" Then continue nursing. It helps to give a baby other things to gnaw on.

### 23. *If I have a breast infection, can I continue to nurse?*

Yes. Studies have shown women who did not stop nursing when they had breast abscesses had much shorter illnesses and were less likely to need surgery. Continued nursing from the affected breast has no adverse effect on the infant.

### 24. *Will birth-control pills affect my milk supply?*

Yes. Studies show birth-control pills directly suppress lactation. If you take the pill, your doctor will probably suggest that you not nurse. However, some women have been successful if they have a good milk supply and if the baby is well-adjusted to the mother's milk before she starts taking the pill.

### 25. *Does breast-feeding act as a contraceptive?*

Women can and do become pregnant while nursing. This is unusual before the first menstrual period if you are nursing completely. Complete breast-feeding may delay the resumption of your menstrual cycle and ovulation. However, if you want to be absolutely sure, use a contraceptive.

### 26. *If I decide not to nurse, how can I prevent my milk from coming in?*

Your doctor will give you pills or a shot to stop the production of your milk. If milk does come in, the pills or shot will ease the discomfort so you can tolerate it.

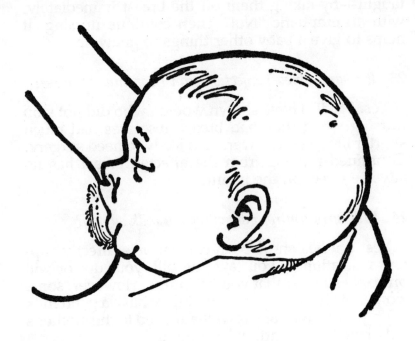

*Position infant's mouth on breast for most-efficient nursing.*

### 27. Are there other ways to relieve pain associated with drying up breasts?

Yes. Ice packs help, and binding the breasts helps somewhat. A tight bra is helpful but not sufficient.

To stop the flow of milk or stop discomfort, use a series of elastic bandages 6 to 8 inches wide as wrap-arounds over your chest and breasts. It is better to empty the breasts completely before applying these bandages.

When you decide to stop nursing, have the baby completely empty the breast. Do not nurse again, even to relieve the discomfort, or you will have to start over each time with the drying-up process.

28. *How can I tell the difference between infection and engorgement of my breasts?*

Engorgement does not cause fever or redness. The pain of engorgement is general throughout the breast. The pain of infection is usually localized and points toward one spot. Engorgement involves both breasts, while infection ordinarily affects only one breast.

---

# SOME TIPS ABOUT NURSING

- Some women have trouble with tender, sore or cracked nipples, but nipples will heal if you persist in nursing your baby.
- The most important preparation is psychological. The most helpful person to talk with is a woman who has successfully nursed her baby.
- Breast-feeding can make a positive contribution to your child's emotional development.
- The woman who is willing to give of herself in breast-feeding is meeting the needs of her growing child.

YOUR BABY NEEDS A BOSOM FRIEND!

---

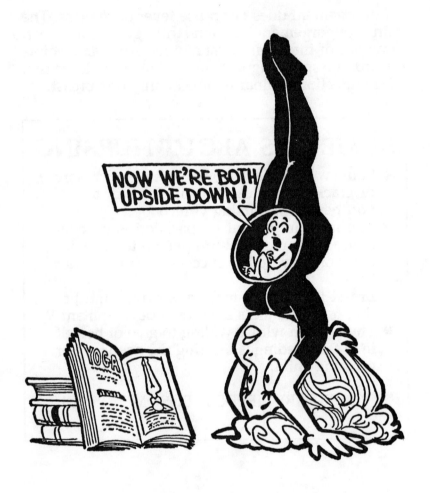

*Come as you are—the baby that is.*

# 26.

# COME AS YOU ARE—
# THE BABY THAT IS

The baby is going to seek the most comfortable position, regardless of whether this makes the trip through the birth canal more difficult. About one in 30 babies will come as a *breech*—either feet or buttocks first.

A few will come out head first but looking upward (sunnyside up) instead of looking down. A rare few come in a position that makes delivery by way of the vagina impossible. Your doctor will be able to recognize and handle these variations.

**1.** *What causes a baby to come in a breech position?*

Sometimes a baby's large head in a small pelvis cannot descend through the birth canal. Because the baby's head does not enter the pelvis, the baby turns and allows the breech, either feet or buttocks, to descend into the pelvis first.

Some women have a pelvis that accommodates a breech position better than a head-first position. For this reason, these women tend to have all of their babies in a breech position.

**2.** *Are there any precautions I should take if my baby is breech?*

Report to your doctor immediately if your bag of waters breaks. There is some increased risk of prolapse of the baby's cord (the cord coming ahead of the baby) so its circulation could be pinched off. Your doctor will want to know as soon as possible if your water breaks before you go into labor.

**3.** *Can a breech baby be turned?*

Yes, in a few cases. But more often the baby returns to the breech position.

**4.** *Is it more difficult to have a baby in the breech position?*

Usually, but with modern pain-relievers, nerve blocks and other anesthesias, you may find little difference. It often means you must work harder to get the baby down far enough in the birth canal for the doctor to deliver him.

**5.** *Is it more dangerous for me to have a breech baby?*

The risk to you is not any greater than for other positions of the baby. However, the risk for the baby is somewhat greater, with a mortality rate of 4% to 6%.

**6.** *Why not have all breech babies by Cesarean operation to avoid risk?*

Some medical centers deliver all breeches by Cesarean. Reliable studies show it is safer to deliver footling and complete breeches, certain premature breeches and large breeches by Cesarean section. Your doctor will decide which method is best for you.

**7.** *If I have a breech birth, will my next baby be breech?*

If you have one breech baby, there is about one chance in five that your next baby will be breech.

8. *Is there a chance of injury to my baby if he is delivered by breech?*

There is a greater chance for injury, but only if there is difficulty in delivery. Your doctor will decide if complications are likely. If there is any question in his mind, he will perform a Cesarean operation. Doctors usually lean heavily toward a Cesarean rather than take chances with you or your baby.

9. *What is a posterior position?*

Most babies are born head first, looking down. However, about 10% are born looking upward, in a posterior position, or at least they come into the birth canal in this position. Certain pelvis shapes favor this position.

Your doctor can tell by examination if your baby is coming in this position. Many "posterior" babies rotate spontaneously during labor and are delivered looking down, which is an easier type of delivery.

Many babies who persist in the posterior position during labor can be turned by the doctor, either with his hand or, if this fails, with delivery instruments. Certain "posterior" babies deliver easily in this posterior position.

10. *Is it more difficult to have a baby in a posterior position?*

Labor is often longer and may be more difficult and painful. The dimensions of the baby's head in this position require more space to allow the head to pass through the pelvis and vagina.

For these reasons, a posterior position may be a more difficult delivery, with a greater tendency for tears in you and injury to the baby. If possible, a posterior position is usually converted by the doctor to an easier "crown-first" position for delivery.

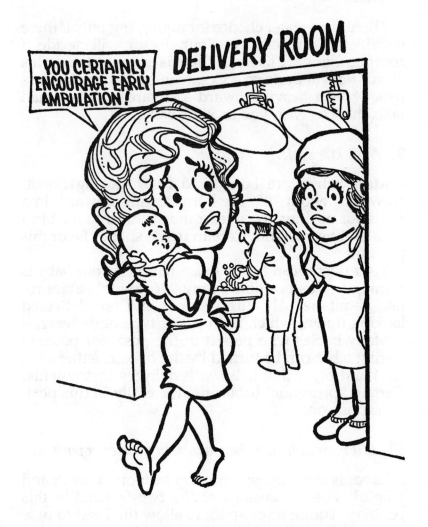

*How soon may I be up and around?*

# 27.

# AFTER MY BABY, THEN WHAT?

For the past several months, anticipation of having your baby has taken precedence over everything else. Would it be a boy or a girl? Would he or she be normal? How would the delivery go? These questions crowded out other considerations—until now. Now that you've had your baby, what's next? What should you expect now and what about the future?

Every new mother faces a different challenge. Every doctor must decide what is best for his particular patient and her needs. Your problems may be different from all others. However, there are still many problems common to nearly all new mothers. Let's discuss a few of them.

1. *How soon may I be up and around?*

This is the day of early ambulation in almost every field of medicine. After a baby, this means "as soon as possible," but may vary according to your labor and delivery and whether complications must be considered. Early ambulation may range from carrying your baby from the delivery room to remaining in bed for several days.

In general, there are few activities you cannot undertake if you do them moderately. Discuss it with your doctor.

## 2. *Will everything fall out when I get up?*

No. This is a remnant from the days when women remained in bed for two to four weeks after delivery. Getting up will not cause anything to fall out or make you bleed excessively if you follow your doctor's direction and do not become overly tired.

## 3. *Will I have afterpains?*

Not all women have afterpains, but these cramplike pains are Nature's attempt to help the uterus contract to stop the bleeding. It is similar to clenching one's hand around a soft tube.

Within a day or two, bleeding is usually under sufficient control so cramps stop. If you have afterpains with the first baby, it is very likely you will have them with subsequent pregnancies. Pains may continue for several days, especially if you nurse your baby.

## 4. *How can my vagina stretch enough to allow a baby to pass through it, then return to normal size after delivery?*

Not only does the vagina have great elasticity, but it is folded into pleats, like an accordion, that flatten out when necessary to accommodate the delivery of the baby. Pregnancy seems to provide additional softening and elasticity of vaginal tissue, which is necessary for the occasion. Tissue tears when a baby is too large or the vagina is too inelastic.

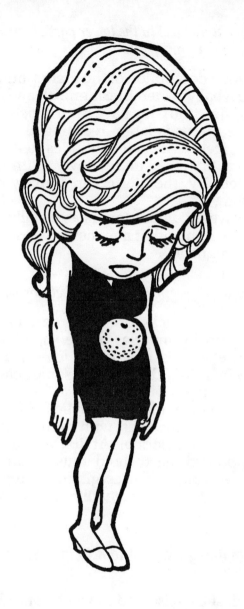

*What's this lump I feel in the lower part of my abdomen?
It's the size of a grapefruit!*

**5.** *What's this lump I feel in the lower part of my abdomen? It's the size of a grapefruit!*

That is a good description of the uterus immediately after having a baby, when the afterbirth and amniotic fluid surrounding the baby have been expelled during delivery. The uterus is large, reaching almost to the navel, and it feels tender. It continues to decrease in size, rapidly at first, then more slowly. Within 10 or 12 days after delivery, the uterus can scarcely be felt in the abdomen.

Within six weeks, your uterus has usually returned to normal size, although it may never be as small as it was before pregnancy.

**6.** *How soon will I begin to look and feel normal again?*

It takes about six weeks for the uterus to return to its normal size and for muscles of the vagina to regain their tone. The process of returning to normal is called *involution*. When it is delayed for some reason, it is called *subinvolution*.

At first, abdominal muscles will be flabby from being overstretched. However, with cautious exercising they slowly return to normal. At first you may wish to wear a support girdle to hold muscles in. As you continue to exercise, muscles gradually regain their former tone, and your figure will return to its former contours.

**7.** *Is there anything I can do to help my organs return to normal faster?*

Rest, modest exercise and a well-balanced diet aid this process. Nursing your baby also seems to speed up involution and makes it more complete.

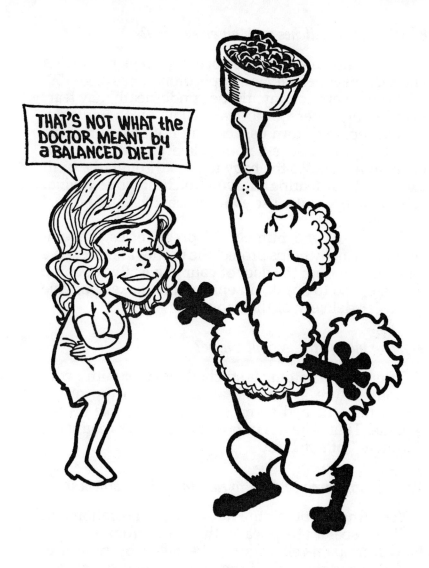

*Is there anything I can do to help my organs return to normal faster?*

## 8. Will I have stitches with an episiotomy?

The incision made by the doctor between the vagina and rectum at delivery is an episiotomy. See page 159. Without an episiotomy, tissues underneath may tear, even though there is no tear visible on the outside. Unless repaired, torn tissues may not heal normally.

Cutting the tissues before delivery (performing an episiotomy) allows the baby to pass through the birth canal without tearing or overstretching your vagina. After delivery, cut muscles are stitched back to normal position.

In spite of the number of pregnancies, an episiotomy usually helps protect the tissues and preserve better support for the floor of your pelvis. By "opening the gate," so to speak, an episiotomy makes possible an easier delivery of the baby.

## 9. How many stitches will I have?

Often an episiotomy is stitched together with a continuous suture in several layers, one on top of the other. It is stitched so no stitches are visible on the outside. Therefore it is impossible for you to count the "number" of stitches.

## 10. Can anything be done to ease the pain of stitches?

Yes. Anesthetic ointments, sprays and lotions, as well as soaks, help ease the pain from stitches. However, pain-relievers can be taken by mouth or given hypodermically if there is undue discomfort.

## 11. How long will I have a vaginal discharge?

Immediately after your baby is born, the discharge consists of pure blood. Gradually this discharge becomes pink, then brown and finally yellow-white. After the first day or two the discharge becomes odorous, yellow-pink and may persist for four to six weeks. During this time the discharge gradually becomes odorless and eventually becomes white in color. The discharge will disappear completely.

12. *Can I douche during this time?*

Discuss it with your doctor first. If all else is normal, he may allow you to douche with a medicinal solution to help diminish the odor and discomfort of the discharge.

13. *I've heard of a tipped uterus. Will being up and around after having a baby cause this?*

No. As far as we know, this is a normal condition for about 25 to 30% of all women. It rarely causes any problems.

14. *How can I avoid after-baby blues?*

After-baby blues are common, and many women have them to some extent. You must realize there is a certain amount of emotional letdown after being emotionally "charged" during your pregnancy.

Avoid excessive fatigue, and ask for help when you need it. If you have problems, there are medicines your doctor can prescribe to prevent as well as treat this condition.

15. *I am worried about my first bowel movement. Will it be painful because of my stitches?*

Usually not. By alternating fecal softeners with large amounts of water, the bowel movement will pass easily and painlessly. However, be sure to drink lots of liquids to give fecal softeners, such as Metamucil, something to work with. Softeners "draw" liquids into the bowel, causing the fecal material to absorb them. In the process, the bowel movement swells up, becomes soft and is easy to pass.

### 16. *What must I avoid during the next few weeks?*

After giving birth, women return to normal surprisingly fast. Check with your doctor because he may have special instructions for you. In general, avoid excessive fatigue. Watch for pain and tenderness in your abdomen, which could mean infection in the pelvic organs. If your breasts become sore, it could mean infection or abscess. Problems with your legs could mean phlebitis. If you begin to pass bright-red blood, notify your doctor immediately!

### 17. *How soon may I resume sexual relations?*

Usually, no earlier than three weeks after delivery, although there are exceptions. Wait until after your 6-week checkup with your doctor. He can assure you that everything has returned to normal. You can also discuss contraception with him.

### 18. *How soon is it possible to become pregnant after having a baby?*

Women have been known to ovulate—release an egg—in the first month after delivery, but usually it takes six weeks. To be safe and sure, use contraceptives.

If you will be using birth-control pills, you may begin taking them immediately after delivery if you are not going to nurse your baby. If you plan to nurse your baby, your doctor may want you to wait until after your lactation is well-established and your baby is getting a good supply of milk before starting you on birth-control pills.

Birth-control pills can cause a decrease in your milk supply. A trace of the ingredients of the pill may also appear in the milk. It is not known what effect this might have on the infant.

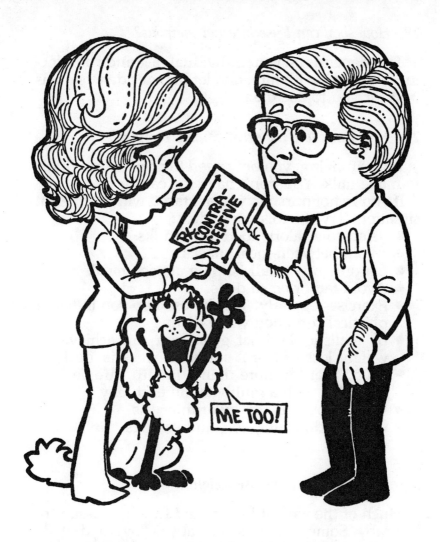

*How soon may I resume sexual relations?*

19. *How soon can I use internal tampons?*

This depends on your individual case and your doctor. Discuss it with him, and let him decide when it is best for you to use them.

20. *How can I lose the extra pounds I gained?*

When nursing, you only need to drink lots of fluids to make milk. You don't have to "eat for two."

If you're not nursing, you are faced with a different situation. Try the following ideas:
- Select low-calorie food and drinks.
- Avoid between-meal snacks.
- Eat only one **small** helping at each meal.
- Avoid fad or crash diets.
- Exercise regularly. This helps keep you in better physical condition while dieting.
- Be realistic, and set goals you can achieve. A weight loss of 1 or 2 pounds a week is ideal.
- If you diet for more than a month, supplement your diet with a multivitamin each day.
- Weigh yourself at regular intervals.
- Calories do count, so count calories.

21. *Why does the baby lose weight at first?*

Much of the weight lost is fluid from the tissues of the baby. Some doctors feel a baby is "overhydrated" before birth and loses some fluid as a normal course of events.

We have also found a baby takes very little nourishment for several days. After he becomes used to eating and is somewhat stabilized, his weight soars rapidly. Birth weight is usually regained in about 10 days.

## 22. Why do they put drops in the baby's eyes?

This is required by law in most states to prevent any chance of gonorrhea from the mother being transferred to the baby's eyes. If untreated, gonorrhea can cause blindness in the baby.

## 23. What about belly bands?

They are used only to appease the mother, but serve no purpose for the baby. Bands do not prevent rupture of the navel in the baby.

## 24. How long before the umbilical cord falls off?

About five to eight days. Ignore it unless the skin around it becomes reddened. Redness around the navel could indicate infection and should be reported to your pediatrician immediately.

# 28.

# EMERGENCY CHILD-BIRTH

Modern transportation has brought nearly every woman within minutes of medical care. Do-it-yourself deliveries are becoming less common. However, campers and trailers have also enabled families to venture far into the hills and deserts. Family boats take them up rivers and across lakes.

Actually, most women who start labor can reach medical facilities if they do not wait too long to make up their minds to go. But you should know what to do in case of an emergency.

Birth is a normal sequence in the normal condition of pregnancy. Even if there are problems, there should be time to get the pregnant woman to a hospital. In the meantime, read the following information.

**Don't Panic!**—If a baby arrives before the mother can get to the hospital, it is nearly always a normal birth. Talk in a calm, reassuring tone of voice to relax and reassure the woman.

**Try to Get Her to the Hospital**—Many women who do not make it to the hospital *could* have made it.

Someone just thought they could not make it. If you see it is impossible to make it to the hospital, call the doctor or an ambulance. Even if late, the doctor can make sure everything is all right, and the mother and baby can be taken to the hospital even after delivery at home.

**Can She Make It to the Hospital?**—If the baby's head is beginning to protrude from the birth canal (vagina), preparation should be made to deliver the baby where the mother is. Jostling of a speeding car at this point only complicates things.

**Make Mother Comfortable**—The safest, most comfortable position is lying down. The mother may feel as though she wants to empty her bladder or bowels, but this could be the uterus and baby bearing down. Have the mother use a bedpan or other basin rather than the toilet.

**Wash Hands Thoroughly**—Use soap and water when you wash your hands, to guard against infection. Do *not* try to wash the mother. It is not necessary to touch her around the vaginal entrance.

**Protect Bed, Floor or Car Seat**—There is usually a large amount of fluid (water and some blood) during a delivery. Provide something to absorb this, such as newspapers, blankets, sheets or towels. Cover anything you use with a clean sheet placed directly under the mother's hips.

**Let Baby Come Naturally**—Nature will usually take care of this. The mother will continue to bear down until the baby is expelled. Do not pull, push, tug or interfere. Let her expel the baby on a clean towel or sheet. If she happens to expel any bowel movement with the baby, cover or remove it so the baby avoids contamination.

**Do I Have to Help With the Delivery?**—Only rarely does the baby need help. In an emergency situation, let the mother expel the baby by herself, without help.

**Do Not Stretch or Pull Cord**—Leave the cord slack, especially while it pulsates. This allows the blood to continue to flow *into* the baby. It is not necessary to cut the cord immediately.

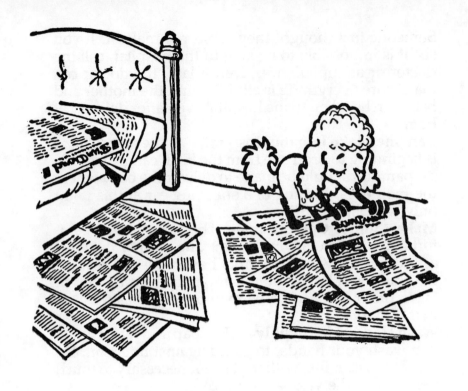

*Protect the bed, floor or car seat.*

If the doctor will arrive within an hour, leave the cord alone. He will take care of this when he arrives. If he cannot be reached, tie the cord *tightly* in two places with a piece of string or strong twine. The closest tie to the baby should be about 6 inches from his navel.

Cut between the two ties with a clean pair of scissors or a knife. There is *no hurry* about cutting the cord.

**If Baby Is Encased in Sac, Break It!**—The sac is usually broken spontaneously during birth. If it is not broken, break it with your fingernail, a pin, the tip of scissors or a knife. Wipe the baby's head. This allows the baby to breathe.

**Wipe Baby's Face**—Wipe the baby's nose and mouth with a clean handkerchief, towel or dishtowel. This is to remove thick mucus and allow the baby to breathe better. Do not use paper tissues that could stick in the nostrils or mouth.

**Place Baby Next to Mother**—The best way to keep a baby warm is to place him in direct contact with the mother's body. If the cord is long enough, the baby can even lie in the mother's arm, next to her breast. If the cord is short, place the baby between the mother's legs after you remove or cover secretions and fluids in the area.

**Cover Baby**—This is for warmth. Use a warm blanket or coat if nothing else is available. Do not cover the baby's head—leave room for him to breathe. Do not let the baby or mother get chilled.

**What About Afterbirth?**—Usually the afterbirth is delivered by itself. When it comes, place it in a basin or newspaper. Do not throw it away. Keep it for the doctor to examine when he arrives. He will want to see if it is complete and make sure none is left in the mother. Do not pull on the cord to deliver the afterbirth.

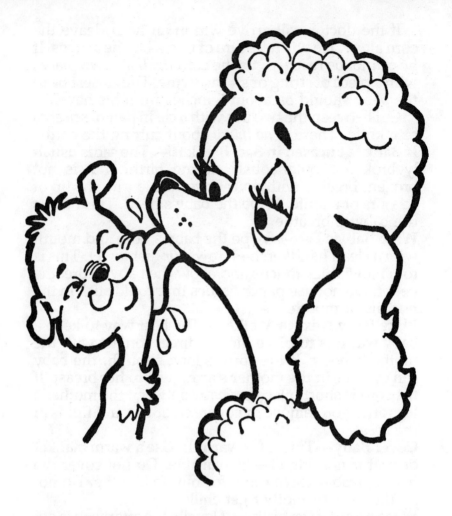

*Wipe baby's face, including nose and mouth, with clean handkerchief, towel or dishtowel.*

**Place Baby at Mother's Breast**—Even if the mother does not intend to nurse her baby, the baby should be placed at her breast to keep the baby warm. When the baby sucks the nipple, it causes the uterus to contract, helping to expel the afterbirth. If the afterbirth has been expelled, sucking causes the uterus to contract to prevent undue bleeding.

**Is It Necessary to Massage Mother's Uterus?**—It is usually wise to gently massage the uterus with a cupped hand after the afterbirth has been expelled. Sometimes the mother can do this herself.

Gentle massage causes the uterus to contract and prevents excessive bleeding. After the uterus clamps down, it will feel firm and will be about the size of a large grapefruit.

After birth of the baby and afterbirth, the following steps should be taken:

- Clean the mother.
- Make her comfortable and warm.
- Do **not** clean the baby. It is better to leave the cheesy coating (vernix) on him at this point.
- Stay with the mother until the doctor arrives.
- If the baby goes to the hospital, place a piece of adhesive tape on his forehead with his mother's name written on it. This assures identification.
- Relax and pat yourself on the back. All three of you made it!

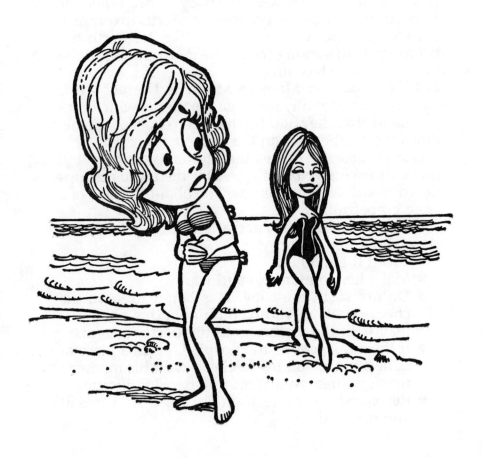

*Is there any way I can avoid stretch marks?*

# 29.

# MISCELLANEOUS QUESTIONS

**1.** *Is there any way I can avoid stretch marks?*

Stretch marks result from rapid overstretching of the skin. Normal skin contains elastic fibers that allow a certain amount of stretching. Some women have more elastic fibers than others.

When the skin is stretched beyond the ability of its elastic fibers, the skin "breaks" and red marks appear. These red marks gradually blanch out and become white, but they never disappear. Fortunately they appear in areas that do not usually show.

Massaging, with or without cocoa butter or any other substance, will not avoid or remove the marks. Avoiding excessive weight gain helps, but often marks depend on the amount of elastic tissue you have inherited. Stretch marks may cause itching.

2. *What happens to my large uterus after my baby is born?*

The uterus is made up of interlacing circular bands of muscle fibers. These fibers contract and squeeze down around the blood vessels so hemorrhage does not occur. The uterus is an adaptable organ that enlarges to accommodate a growing pregnancy, then decreases in size when your baby and afterbirth are delivered.

3. *Is there any reason I can't take a tub bath during pregnancy?*

It was thought that tub baths might cause infection if water reached the vagina and cervix. This has been disproved, and a pregnant woman is allowed to shower or bathe as she pleases any time during pregnancy, until she goes into labor. This does not apply to hot tubs or spas where water temperatures may be extremely high. It is best to avoid hot tubs and spas during pregnancy.

A daily bath using a mild soap is advisable. Be careful to avoid slipping or falling on the wet surface while getting in or out of the tub or shower. Use a rubber mat or non-slip strips on the bottom of your tub or shower stall. Some doctors prefer that you shower if the bag of waters has broken or if there is any bleeding.

4. *In premature babies, does a 7-month baby do better than an 8-month baby?*

No. This is an old wives' tale. In general, the more mature the baby, the better his chances of survival.

5. *Should I avoid contact with animals while pregnant?*

There are several diseases harmful to unborn babies that a pregnant woman can contract from pets, especially from handling a pet's feces or litterbox. If you own a pet, discuss precautions with your doctor.

**6.** *I've noticed many pregnant women have swollen legs and ankles. Is this normal?*

Nearly 80% of all pregnant women have some sort of swelling. Swelling is at least average and very common. Some swelling can be avoided by forcing fluids and avoiding *excess* salt in the diet. However, do not go on a salt-free diet while you are pregnant.

If swelling becomes so severe that you can't tolerate it, your doctor may prescribe diuretic pills. However, they must be carefully controlled and should never be taken without the doctor's permission—especially during pregnancy!

If the swelling is accompanied by elevated blood pressure or albumin in the urine, it is more serious. Together, these are the signs of toxemia of pregnancy. A section on *Toxemia of Pregnancy* begins on page 121.

**7.** *What about dark blotches across my cheeks and forehead?*

This is often called the *mask of pregnancy* by some and *liver spots* by others, although blotches have nothing to do with the liver. Blotches are common, especially in brunettes, and there is no way to avoid them. Sunlight tends to make them more intense and noticeable.

Marks gradually fade after pregnancy but have a tendency to persist in some individuals. Some blanching preparations help make blotches less conspicuous.

**8.** *Why does my skin feel so tight?*

Your skin is stretching, but it is common to feel as though it is tightly stretched during pregnancy. Massage your skin gently with lotion. It will not prevent stretch marks, but it will make you feel better.

**9.** *Will I have problems with my teeth during pregnancy?*

Not particularly, but visit your dentist to have any necessary dental work done. Good dental hygiene and a well-balanced diet are your best assurance of a healthy mouth.

If you vomit, be sure to rinse your mouth often to avoid corrosive action of stomach acid on the enamel of your teeth.

**10.** *What can I do to relieve itching of my breasts, abdomen and hip area, especially where there are stretch marks?*

There are many good lotions and even more theories about cures for this. First, make sure your soap is non-allergenic. Rinse your skin thoroughly after bathing or washing.

One of the best non-allergenic preparations is rose water mixed with glycerine. Many companies make this kind of lotion or cream. If you don't want to use this, choose a lotion or cream that agrees with you. For best results, apply lotion or cream to damp skin.

**11.** *Why do I have large veins in my legs? Will they disappear after pregnancy?*

Due to loss of tone in the walls of the veins, they become stretched. This allows blood to "puddle," especially in the legs. These veins become enlarged and engorged as they literally sag with blood.

Veins also become unsightly. It may be one of the first things you notice when you become pregnant.

Varicose veins are usually hereditary. Temporary relief may be found by elevating legs as much as possible. Be sure your legs are higher than your pelvis.

If lying on a couch, drape your feet over the back of the couch. When you're in bed, you can place two pillows under your legs. Another method is to turn a kitchen chair upside down, place a pillow on the back of it, then lie flat on the floor and drape your legs over the chair back.

If your doctor suggests elastic stockings, do not confuse these with support hose. Elastic stockings must be specially fitted to you and should be put on before you get out of bed. Support hose, by contrast, are sold in stores in small, medium and large sizes. Either or both may be effective.

Ordinarily, varicose veins disappear after pregnancy. If they persist and are severe, they can be corrected by surgery. Surgery on varicose veins is best deferred until *after* pregnancy.

12. *Does it matter how I stand, sit or lie, as far as my baby is concerned?*

No, as long as you are comfortable. The baby seems to adjust accordingly.

13. *Is there anything I do that could "mark" my baby?*

There is nothing we know of that will mark your baby. It is best to regard pregnancy as a normal state of being and continue to live as though you were not pregnant.

14. *Is my baby affected by my thoughts and feelings?*

If you are excited or afraid, the baby might be more active in the uterus at that time. But there is no evidence such an effect is lasting, as far as the baby is concerned.

15. *What are hemorrhoids? My mother said I might have them.*

Hemorrhoids are varicose veins of the rectum. Like other varicose veins, hemorrhoids are common during pregnancy. This is not serious. Try the following suggestions:
- Develop a regular bowel habit—same time each day.
- Drink plenty of liquids, preferably two quarts a day.

- Avoid straining.
- If necessary, use a stool softener.
- Honey may prevent constipation in some women. Use it in cooking or mix it with warm water or milk and drink it at night.
- Elevate your feet, such as on a foot stool, while sitting on the toilet.
- Keep the rectal area clean and dry. A cool astringent pack often gives temporary relief.
- Anesthetic ointments, prescribed by your doctor, may relieve pain and itching.
- Report bleeding from the rectum to your doctor immediately.

16. *I want to feel beautiful while I'm pregnant, but I don't know what to do. Can you help?*

Pregnancy is a very special time for you and your growing baby. Feeling good about yourself is important. One good book, also published by HPBooks, is *Pregnant & Beautiful! How to Eat Right, Stay Fit & Look Great*. It has hundreds of beauty and fashion tips to help you look and feel beautiful all through pregnancy.

# 30.

# CONTRACEPTION

Aside from complete abstinence or surgical removal of the organs, there is no 100% effective method of birth control or contraception. Birth-control pills, more than any other form of contraception, are close to 100% effective. We will discuss many forms of contraception in this section.

**RHYTHM METHOD**

The method known as the rhythm method or safe period is widely used, especially by members of certain religious groups who do not wish to use artificial means of birth control. More accurate would be the title "relatively" safe period, for the average woman's cycle is unpredictable. Many women will occasionally be unsafe, even when, according to the calendar, they should be safe from conception.

The rhythm method is based on two theories. The first is the average woman ovulates, or gives off an egg from her ovary every 28 days. The second theory is ovulation occurs about 14 days before her next expected menstrual period begins. Therefore, the fertile, or unsafe, time for a 28-day-cycle person is 14 days before her next expected menstrual period and 14 days after her last menstrual period.

If a woman has a 35-day cycle, her most fertile time is still 14 days before her next expected menstrual period. But it now would be 21 days after the first day of her last menstrual period. The farther from this fertile time one departs, the safer the time becomes.

In a 28-day-cycle woman, the safest time is just before and just after a menstrual period. Allow three or four days on either side of the ovulation time as fertile. Any remaining days should be relatively safe.

One method of determining the safe period is to record your temperature the first thing in the morning, preferably at the same time each day. Watch for a rise of 0.4 to 0.8 of a degree at the fertile time. This same method may be used to determine the optimum time for conception, as well as contraception.

## CONDOM OR SHEATH

Your husband may use a condom, rubber sheath or prophylactic to contain the semen and sperm during intercourse to prevent conception. This method is effective and especially adapted to the couple in which the wife is unable or unwilling to use contraception.

Check the sheath first to be sure there are no leaks. It should be placed on the penis before coitus begins. Many couples do not realize one cause of unexpected pregnancy is that sperm remains in the male urethra without ejaculation.

Until the recent precautions that have become necessary because of sexually transmitted diseases, especially AIDS, herpes and chlamydia, condoms were regarded as awkward and outdated. However, since there is no cure for either AIDS or herpes, the condom has become a most important part of prevention of the spread of STD's.

Since 40% of all condoms are sold to women, we have included the following instructions in their use, and also some ready answers when their at-risk partner hedges or even refuses to use a condom.

# HOW TO USE A CONDOM

## How to Buy Condoms

DO buy a supply of latex, reservoir (nipple) end lubricated type condoms. They're available in different colors, textures and sometimes in two different sizes. A good quality condom is the most important feature for safer sex.

DO check expiration date on outer package.

DO store in a cool dry place.

DO carry a condom with you at all times.

DON'T buy condoms made of any material other than latex (only latex prevents passage of harmful germs).

DON'T buy old (outdated) condoms.

DON'T store condoms in hot glove compartments of car. Heat can damage the condom.

DON't carry in hip wallet for long periods of time—this shortens shelf life.

DON'T be shy about buying condoms—remember, 40% are sold to women.

## How to Put the Condom On:

DO remove rolled condom from package.

DO roll condom down on penis as soon as it is hard, *before* you start to make love.

DO leave 1/4—1/2 inch extra space at time of condom to catch the ejaculate if the condom has no nipple.

DON't unroll condom; instead carefully roll on all the way toward the base of penis.

DON'T put condom on only as your husband is ready to enter—it may be too late. Drops of semen may ooze from the uncovered penis before ejaculation and may infect or impregnate you.

DON'T twist or tear condom —this will damage its effectiveness

**How to Take a Condom off:**
DO hold the condom at the rim; remove soon after ejaculation.
DO keep used condom away from your husband's genitals and other areas of the body.
DON'T let penis go soft inside vagina—condom may drop off, and protection is lost.
DON't tug to pull condom off—it may tear.

**How to Take a Condom Off:**
DON'T allow semen to spill on your hands or body.
DO wash hands or body parts if contact occurs.
DO wrap condom in tissue and dispose of safely.
DON'T allow semen to come in contact with a skin break, cut, or open wound.

**Special Points to Remember**
If you buy unlubricated condoms, you may need to buy a lubricant. Use only water soluble lubricants such as spermicidal jelly or water.

Don't use oil-based lubricants such as petroleum jelly or vegetable oil with latex condoms, since they can damage the condom.

Never use a condom more than once.

Correct use of condoms increases comfort, and promotes a sense of security in having safer sex.

SEXUAL ABSTINENCE IS THE ONLY SURE WAY TO PREVENT PREGNANCY AND SEXUALLY TRANSMITTED DISEASES, INCLUDING AIDS. IF YOU DECIDE TO HAVE SEX, CORRECT USE OF A CONDOM WILL HELP TO PROTECT YOURSELF AND YOUR HUSBAND AGAINST THESE RISKS.

## HOW TO TALK ABOUT CONDOMS WITH SOMEONE WHO IS RESISTANT, DEFENSIVE, OR MANIPULATIVE:

**If he says:**
"I know I'm clean (disease-free)."

**You can say:**
"Thanks for telling me. As far as I know, I'm disease-free, too "

"I haven't had sex with anyone in X months."

"But I'd like to use a condom—since either of us could have an infection and not know it."

● "I'm a virgin."

"I'm not. This way we'll both be protected."

● "I can't feel a thing when I wear a condom; it's like wearing a raincoat in the shower."

"Even if you lose some sensation, you'll still have plenty left."

"I'll lose my erection by the time I stop and put it on."

"I'll help you put it on— that'll help you keep it."

"By the time you put it on, I'm out of the mood."

"Maybe so, but we feel strongly enough for each other to stay in the mood."

- "Condoms are unnatural and a total turnoff."

  "Please let's try to work this out—an infection isn't so great either. So let's give the condom a try. Or maybe we can look for alternatives."

- "What kind of alternative?"

  "Maybe we'll just pet or postpone sex for awhile."

- "This is an insult. Do you think I'm disease-ridden?"

  "I didn't say or imply that. I care for you, but in my opinion, it's best to use a condom."

- "I love you! Would I give you an infection?"

  "Not intentionally. But many people don't know they're infected. That's why this is best for both of us right now."

- "Just this once."

  "Once is all it takes."

- "I don't have a condom with me."

  "I do" or "Then let's satisfy each other without intercourse."

- "You carry a condom around with you? You were planning to seduce me!"

  "I always carry one with me because I care about myself. I have one with me tonight because I care about us both."

## DIAPHRAGM WITH JELLY

A diaphragm used with jelly or cream is an effective, harmless method of contraception. The diaphragm must be fitted by a physician, and it should be combined with a jelly or contraceptive cream and left in place a minimum of 8 to 12 hours after intercourse.

## JELLY OR CREAM

Spermicidal jellies and creams may be used without a diaphragm, but their effectiveness is decreased. It is not only the diaphragm that prevents conception, but the spermicidal effect of the jelly or cream.

The diaphragm ensures the jelly or cream will be held in place. However, many women have used only spermicidal jellies and creams alone for many years and swear by their effectiveness.

## FOAMS

With the advent of new packaging, it was natural that jellies and creams would be placed in containers with compressed air. This product is the one that is most widely used. The effectiveness of foam approximates that of jelly or cream, but it may be more convenient to use. Like the diaphragm, jelly, cream or condom must be used before intercourse begins. Postcoital douching is best delayed until 8 to 12 hours after intercourse.

## SUPPOSITORIES

These small pellets of low-melting-point preparations can be inserted into the vagina prior to coitus. They melt and provide protection equivalent to jellies, creams and foams.

## SPONGES

There is now a sponge available that contains spermicidal jelly. So far, it has proved to be effective and easy to use.

## DOUCHES

The post-coital douche is as old as the contraceptive idea and has been effective for many women. However, it carries a fair risk of pregnancy and should not be relied on as much as other methods.

Various preparations have been used with testimonials for all. In general, we cannot recommend these with great assurance.

## COITUS INTERRUPTUS

Coitus interruptus, or withdrawal, is the oldest method of contraception known to man. Bascially, the man withdraws his penis from the vagina prior to ejaculation of sperm, thus avoiding conception.

Although many couples find this method satisfactory, there are some disadvantages. First, it places a strain on what should be an unstrained relationship. Both the husband and wife may worry about his withdrawing soon enough to prevent any sperm from entering the vagina. Second, it prevents the husband from completing the normal sexual act. At the height of physical ecstasy, he must suddenly withdraw and interrupt this very special moment of shared pleasure.   There is considerable evidence to indicate a damaging psychological effect of coitus interruptus; in a number of men, it is alleged to have caused impotence. Interruption may also prevent the woman from achieving her normal climax because withdrawal may come as she is beginning, or is in the middle of, her orgasm.

Third, sperm may be found in the normal male urethra that could escape into the vagina before ejaculation of the sperm and cause conception.

## INTRAUTERINE DEVICES

Intrauterine devices (IUDs) have been used for many years but are now frowned on by the medical profession. The only approved IUD is the progestasert, but after women and physicians read through several pages of warnings about the device, both usually agree to alternate methods.

## ORAL CONTRACEPTIVES

To better inform our patients of oral contraception, we have prepared this fairly short statement for them to read and sign before we prescribe any oral contraception. We suggest that you read this statement carefully before you take oral contraception.

# INFORMED CONSENT/
## ORAL CONTRACEPTIVES

Before you give your consent be sure you understand the benefits and risks of oral contraceptives. If you have any questions as you read, we will be happy to discuss them.

I am aware that oral contraceptives can be close to 98-99% effective if I take them consistently and correctly. I understand that the progestin-only pills (Mini-Pills) are 97% effective if taken correctly.

I understand that the main advantage of oral contraceptives is prevention of pregnancy. In addition, some women experience the following *benefits* from using oral contraceptives:

- decreased menstrual cramps and decreased menstrual bleeding
- more regular menstrual bleeding
- decreased ovulation pain
- improvement of acne
- less risk of developing ovarian and/or endometrial cancer
- less risk of developing benign breast tumors or ovarian cysts
- less risk of acute pelvic inflammatory disease
- less iron deficiency anemia

I am aware of these *major risks* of birth control pills, many of which can be temporary or life threatening:

- blood clots of the legs or lungs
- stroke or heart attack
- gallbladder disease
- rare type of liver tumor
- hypertension which is usually reversible
- death from heart attacks or strokes
- spotting between periods
- breast tenderness
- weight gain
- headaches
- depression
- mood changes
- fatigue
- changes in sex drive
- darkening of the skin on the face
- increased acne
- missed periods
- decreased menstrual bleeding
- nausea

I am aware that cardiovascular risks are extremely rare and occur primarily in a small subgroup of women who use the pill. Women most at risk of developing cardiovascular side effects are those that have other characteristics that serve to increase their risk. I am aware that my risk is increased if I have any of the following risk factors:

Smoking: Women over 30 who smoke 15 cigarettes a day are at increased risk.

Other health problems such as: hypertension, diabetes, a history of heart or vascular disease.

Women who have a family history of diabetes or heart attack under the age of 50.

I have been informed to watch out for the following *Pill Danger Signals* and to contact my physician at once if I develop one of these problems. These could be warnings of serious or even life-threatening illness:

- abdominal pain (severe), yellowing of the skin.
- chest pain (severe), cough, shortness of breath.
- headaches (severe), dizziness, weakness or numbness.
- eye problems (vision loss or blurring).
- severe leg pain, redness or swelling.

I have been instructed on how to use the birth control pills.

I have been given the opportunity to discuss alternate methods of birth control and feel that oral contraceptives are my choice for birth control.

I have been given the opportunity to ask questions about oral contraceptives.

My questions have been answered to my satisfaction.

NAME _____

WITNESS _____

DATE _____

COMMENTS _____

_____

_____

_____

## SPECIAL NEEDS

If you have, or have had, special health problems, such as migraine headaches, mental depression, fibroids of the uterus, heart or kidney disease, asthma, high blood pressure, diabetes or epilepsy, tell your doctor. He may wish to make sure the pill is suitable for you by doing special tests. Some conditions may be made worse by the use of oral contraceptives.

Report to your doctor any unusual swelling, skin rash, yellowing of the skin or eyes or severe depression.

There are women who should never use oral contraceptives. They include: those with tendencies toward blood-clotting disorders, women who have cancer of the breast or womb, and women with serious liver conditions or undiagnosed vaginal bleeding when cancer has not been ruled out should not take oral contraceptives. It is comforting to know your doctor can recommend other methods of birth control.

## SUMMARY

Oral contraceptives, when taken as directed, are extraordinarily effective drugs. As with other medicine, side effects are possible. The most serious is abnormal blood clotting. Serious problems are relatively rare, and the majority of women can use the pill safely and effectively.

See your physician regularly. Discuss with him any concerns you may have about the use of the pill, and report any special problems that may arise.

As a contraceptive, the pill is almost 100% effective. Only rarely does a conception occur when the pill is used as prescribed. It is convenient and is usually well-tolerated, although sometimes there are a few side effects.

The pill prevents conception by preventing ovulation. It keeps a woman from giving off an egg. However, forgetting to take the pill may allow ovulation to occur.

Ordinarily, one day's dose can be missed without ovulation and conception occurring. However, when a pill is forgotten, two pills should be consumed the following day. Failure to take several pills is usually followed by spotting or bleeding within two to three days. This is a built-in alarm to alert the woman to start taking her pills again and to use an additional method of protection for the next week.

The pill prevents ovulation, and thus prevents pregnancy. Women may experience side effects such as nausea, fatigue, weight gain, change in pigmentation of the skin, loss of libido and loss of pleasant disposition. Occasionally some side effects are more serious.

Many women experience no unpleasant side effects. Among those who do, most who persist in taking the pill, overcome all discomfort. Usually any discomfort is more than compensated for by the peace of mind women find in safety from conception.

There are other important things you should know about the pill, and these may best be handled in question-and-answer form.

1. *Why are there so many different doses, strengths and combinations of birth-control pills?*

Because everyone reacts differently to a given birth-control pill. For this reason, it's best for your doctor to prescribe the proper pill for you.

2. *If I forget a pill, will I get pregnant?*

You certainly may be vulnerable, especially if you miss several pills early in any pill cycle. If you miss several pills, expect to spot or even start a flow. Take two pills a day for two or three days, and use an additional method of contraception for at least a week while you continue your pill schedule. If you have any questions, call your doctor.

**3.** *Why would I spot if I didn't miss a day with my pills?*

This does not mean you are or could become pregnant. Sometimes this happens, especially during the first month of taking the pill. Continue taking your pills as directed. If spotting persists for more than two months, consult your doctor. He may change the dosage of your pill.

**4.** *What if I miss a menstrual period, even though I have not missed a pill?*

Occasionally this happens to women who are taking the pill. Continue to take your pills as scheduled to protect you from pregnancy. If you miss two menstrual periods, consult your doctor.

**5.** *Should I take the pill at any special time of day?*

It does not really matter when you take the pill, but take it at about the same time each day. Some women starting the pill, find they tolerate it better if it is taken with a meal, especially the evening dinner.

**6.** *Am I protected from pregnancy as soon as I begin taking the pill in the first cycle?*

If you begin taking them on the fifth day of menstrual flow, you will receive the full benefit of the medication for the month following. However, if you begin your first cycle of pills after day five, use an additional method of contraception for one week. This extra protection will not be necessary after your first cycle of the pill.

**7.** *Does the pill cause women who take it to become pregnant later in life? Can taking the pill postpone menopause?*

No. This is not possible.

8. *Would there be any serious harm done if a child accidentally took a birth-control pill?*

No. However, a child may get nauseous and vomit. If a child does take one, check with your local poison control center or your pediatrician.

9. *Do birth-control pills cause twins, triplets and other multiple births?*

No. Fertility pills do.

10. *Will the pill cause miscarriage if taken inadvertently by a pregnant woman?*

No.

11. *How soon after my baby is born can I start taking the pill?*

There are different circumstances, so discuss it with your doctor and follow his directions.

12. *Can I switch from one brand of birth-control pills to another?*

Yes. However, because of varying doses, do so only under your doctor's direction.

13. *How long may I continue to use the pill?*

If you smoke, stop at least by age 35. If you don't smoke, stop by age 40.

# ABOUT THE AUTHORS

Lindsay R. Curtis, M.D., a retired physician from Ogden, Utah, obtained his B.A. degree from the University of Utah and his M.D. from the University of Colorado School of Medicine. He is a Fellow of the American College of Obstetrics and Gynecology, a Diplomate of the American Board of Obstetrics and Gynecology and was an Assistant Clinical Professor of Obstetrics and Gynecology at the University of Utah College of Medicine. He was also educational consultant for the Utah Division of the American Cancer Society.

Dr. Curtis is past-president of the Utah Obstetrical and Gynecological Society and past-president of the Ogden Surgical Society. He has authored several books, including "About My Daughter, Doctor," "Feminine and Fit," "Solving Sex Problems in Marriage" and "Sensible Sex." He was also the author of a syndicated medical column, "For Women Only," carried in many newspapers in the United States, Canada, Europe and South America.

Yvonne Coroles, R.N., is the Director of Nursing at Dixie Medical Center, St. George, Utah. Previously she was head Nurse of Labor and Delivery at McKay-Dee Hospital in Ogden, Utah, where she taught a course in Childbirth Education to expectant parents for more than 20 years. Many of the questions in this book were developed from that course. She has also lectured widely and written articles on pregnancy and related subjects.

# INDEX

**A**

Abdomen
  itching 206
  tightening 145
Abdominal breathing 34
Abdominal pain 45, 91
Abortion 55, 82, 108
Acquired Immune Deficiency Syndrome (AIDS) 105, 106
After-baby blues 191
Afterbirth 17, 19, 21, 22, 48, 57, 58, 60, 70, 89, 108, 114, 128, 139, 151, 161, 162, 188
Afterpains 186
Albumin in urine 121, 205
Alcohol 171
Amniocentesis 26, 74, 129
Amniotic fluid 14, 17, 19, 26, 48, 139, 188,
  excessive 19
Analgesic 42
Anemia 41
Anesthesia 26, 151, 152, 158, 182, 190
Animals, care of 204
*Anovulatory* 14
Antibiotics 62, 104
Anticoagulants 45
Antihistamines 62
Antithyroid drugs 45
Anxiety 7
Appendicitis 45, 91
Asphyxia 21
*Atelectasis* 29

**B**

Baby blues 191
Baby
  birth weight 194
  dehydrated 22
  due date 32
  eye color 29
  premature 204
  size 21
  weight 137, 139
Backache 46, 96, 98, 143, 145
Bag of waters 14, 19, 85, 91, 148, 158, 182
Basic food groups 141
Bathing 46, 204
Bicycling 64
Birth control 85, 209-223
Birth defects 17, 19, 24, 26, 58, 62, 78, 79, 82, 129
  central nervous system 79
  hearing loss 79
  heart 62, 79
  hemophilia 26
  limb 62
  purple birthmarks 82
  sex-linked 26
  spina bifida 17
  stunted growth 82
  vision loss 79
Birth weight 22
Birth-control pills 14, 39, 62, 104, 177, 192, 217-223
  milk supply 177
Birthing room 152, 153
Bladder 36, 91
  infection 91

Bleeding 83, 85, 110, 114, 115, 119, 148, 161, 162
  abdominal pain 115
  atony 162
  causes 115
  laceration 162
  painless 114
  pieces of afterbirth 162
  tears 162
  uterine 83
Bloated 34, 51
Blood pressure 121, 122, 205
Blood transfusion 119
Bloody discharge from vagina 89
Bloody show 148
Blurring of vision 121
Bottle-feeding 166
Bowel movement, first 191
Bowling 63
Braxton-Hicks contractions 146
Breast infection, nursing 175
Breast milk
  alcohol 171
  amount of 169
  chocolate 171
  laxatives 171
  pumping 169
  spicy food 171
Breast-feeding 13, 164-179
  as contraceptive 177
Breasts 7, 13, 14, 32, 34, 48, 139, 165, 166, 173, 177, 179, 192, 206
Breathing, abdominal 34
Breech birth
  anesthesia 182
  causes 181
  pain relief 182
  precautions 182

**C**

Calcium 46
Calories 50, 142
Cancer 62, 132, 173
Carbohydrates 48, 139
Cesarean operation 19, 24, 26, 27, 119, 122, 133, 135, 136, 153, 173, 182, 183
Charley horse 46
Chills 91
*Chlamydia* 100-103
Chocolate 171
Clotting defects 163
Coitus 24, 83
Coitus interruptus 216
Cold tablets 62
Colostrum 14, 165
Conception 24, 58, 117
Condoms 210-214
Contraception 209-223
Constipation 36, 45, 91, 96
Contraception 192, 211-223
Contractions 83, 111, 113, 114, 143, 146, 149, 153
Cramping 110, 111, 143, 145, 186
Cramps 46
Cysts 8

**D**
D and C 111
Danger signs of pregnancy 89-93
  abdominal pain 91
  bleeding 89
  bloody discharge from vagina 89
  burning urination 91
  chills and fever 91
  headache 91
  nausea and vomiting 91
  reduced amount of urine 91
  sudden gush of water 91
  swelling 91
  vision problems 91
Dark blotches 205
Delivery 22, 26, 29, 45, 74, 86, 88, 108, 126, 128, 137, 151, 152, 153, 155, 158, 161, 162, 163, 182, 183
Demerol anesthesia 151
Diabetes 91, 104
Diaphragm 215
Diet 46, 49, 51, 137, 188
  sample 49
  well-balanced 188
Digestion 34, 51, 96, 152
Dilatation 146
Douche 100, 216
Down's Syndrome 26
Drugs 45, 57, 58, 151
Dry birth 19, 158

**E**
Ectopic pregnancy 117, 119
Egg 8, 10, 19
Electrolyte balance 53, 55
Embryo 19, 27, 32, 58, 60
Emergency childbirth 196-201
Emotions 13, 39, 51, 53, 96
Engorgement of breasts 7, 32, 34
Epidural-block anesthesia 151
Episiotomy 159, 190
*Erythroblastosis fetalis* 26, 71, 75
Erythroblasts 71, 72
Estrogen 62, 100
Exchange transfusions 74
Exercise 46, 98, 188
Exercises, breast 32

**F**
Fainting 42, 98, 118
Fallopian tubes 7, 8, 117, 135
False labor 128, 146
False pregnancy 8
Fatigue 7, 39, 86, 95, 192
Fats and oils 49, 139
Fertility 10
Fertilization 8, 31
Fertilized egg 8, 10, 117, 126
Fetal monitoring 153
Fetal position 22
Fetus 21, 22, 27, 48, 58, 60, 78, 114, 129, 131, 145
  bowel movements 21
  breathing 22
  development 27
  digestion 21
  drops 145
  growth 48
  heart 60
  hiccups 22
  legs 60
  nervous system 60

  visual system 60
Fever 91
Fontanels 22
Forceps delivery 128
Formula 169, 171
Fraternal twins 126, 128

**G**
Gall bladder 45, 91
German measles, see *Rubella*
Glands 32
Glasses 42
Golf 63
Gonorrhea 100, 101, 194
Gynecological exam 7

**H**
HI test 78
Headache 42, 121
Heartburn 34
Hemorrhoids 207, 208
Herpes 104, 106
Hiccups 22
High blood pressure 91
Home delivery 153
Hormones 13, 21, 36, 39, 45, 51, 60, 62, 108
Horseback riding 64
Hydramnios 17
Hydrochloric acid 53
Hyperimmune gamma globulin 72, 75
Hysterectomy 136

**I**
Identical twins 126, 128
Immune response 70, 129
Impaired immune response 129
Implantation 58
Indigestion 34, 96
Infection 26, 99, 108, 148, 192
Intercourse 83, 85, 86
Intrauterine device (IUDs) 119, 217
Intravenous fluids 53
Involution 171, 188
Itching 101, 206

**L**
Labor 18, 45, 89, 91, 107, 108, 111, 113, 114, 135, 143, 145, 146, 148, 152, 158, 183
Labor pains 143, 158
Labor
  difficult 163
  eating 152
  false 128, 146
  length 149
  second stage 155
  stages 149
  third stage 161, 162
Lamaze 151, 152
Laxatives 36, 45, 62, 96, 171
Libido 85, 86
Liquids 55
Liver spots 205
Losing weight 194
Lunar months 21, 31

**M**
Mask of pregnancy 205
Massage, back 46
Massaging uterus 162

Measles 78
Meconium 17, 21
Medicines 34, 45, 57, 62, 96, 101, 104
   antibiotics 62
   antihistamines 62
   aspirin 62
   cold tablets 62
   laxatives 62
   over-the-counter 62
   pain pills 62
   sedatives 62
   tranquilizers 62
   weight-control pills 62
Menstrual cycle 31, 148, 177, 213
Menstrual period 5, 7, 8, 14, 24, 31, 32, 58, 80, 110, 118, 131, 143, 177,
Midwives 152
Minerals 49, 139
Miscarriage 64, 83, 86, 89, 107, 108, 110, 111, 114
   bleeding 110
   cramping 110
   warning signs 110
*Moniliasis* 104
Monitoring 153
   external 153
   fetal pulse 153
   internal 153
Morning sickness, see *Nausea*
Multiple births 125, 126

**N**
Nausea 7, 53, 91, 51-55
   abortion 55
   electrolyte balance 53, 55
   foods 53, 55
   hydrochloric acid 53
   intravenous fluids 53
   liquids 55
   meals 55
   sedation 53
   vitamins 55
   weight loss 53
Nipple-rolling exercise 165
Nipple
   care 165
   stimulation 88
Nisentil anesthesia 151
Nursing 13, 34, 164-179, 188, 194
   as contraceptive 177
   baby teething 175
   breasts 164
   lack of milk 164
   preparing to 164
   sore nipples 164
   starting 175
   tips 179
   twins 169
   weight loss 164
Nutrition 137, 141

**O**
Oligohydramnios 17
Oral contraceptives 217-223
Orgasm 86
Over-the-counter drugs 62
Ovulation 14, 24, 31, 177, 192, 211

**P**
Pain pills 62

Pain relief 42, 62, 98, 151, 182
Pains, labor 143, 158
Pap smear 7
Passive immunity 71, 72
Pelvic exam 7, 41, 115, 148
Pelvic Inflammatory Disease (PID) 100
Pelvic measurements 41
Penile discharge 101
Physical changes 13
Placenta 17, 19, 21, 22, 48, 57, 58, 60, 70, 108, 114, 128, 139, 161, 162, 188
Placenta, premature separation 115
*Placenta previa* 108, 114, 135
Placental barrier 57
Posterior position 183
Posture 34, 46, 98
Precoital douche
   acid 24
   alkaline 24
Pregnancy danger signs 89-93
Pregnancy changes 8, 13
Pregnancy complications 137
Pregnancy discomforts 95
Pregnancy, false 8
Pregnancy signs
   anxiety 7
   discoloration of skin 7
   engorgement of breasts 7
   fatigue 7
   frequent urination 7
   morning sickness 7
   soreness of breasts 7
Pregnancy test 5, 8
   blood 5
   urine 5, 8
Premature baby 107, 111, 175
   nursing 175
Premature birth 128
Premature separation of placenta 115
Progesterone 100
Prolapse of umbilical cord 182
Protein 48, 139
Pudendal-block anesthesia 151

**Q**
Quadruplets 126
Quickening 8
Quintuplets 126

**R**
Rh D-factor 69
Rh-factor 41, 69-75
   immune response 70
Rh-negative 69
Rh-sensitization 71, 72, 75
RhoGam 72, 75
Rhythm method 209
Rubella 41, 58, 77-82
   birth defects 79, 82
   blood test 80
   diagnosis 78
   immunization 80
   incubation period 77
   HI test 78
   symptoms 77
   treatment 78
   vaccine 79
Rubella encephalitis 82
Running 67

**S**

Second stage of labor 155
Sedation 53
Sedatives 62
Sex, determining 24, 26
Sexually Transmitted Diseases (STDs) 99-100
Shock 118
Showing 113, 114
Skiing 64
Skin discoloration 7
Soft spots 22
Sonograms 125, 129-132
Soreness of breasts 7
Speculum 7
Sperm 8, 10
Spermicidal jelly or cream 215
Spicy food 171
Spina bifida 17
Spinal anesthesia 151, 158
Sponges 215
Stages of labor 149
Stairs 64
Sterility 108
Sterilization 135
Stitches, pain 190, 191
Streptomycin 45
Stretch marks 203
Subinvolution 188
Suppositories 215
Swelling 91, 121, 122, 128, 205
Swimming 63, 67

**T**

ampons 192
Teenage pregnancies 48
Teeth, problems 206
Tennis 63
Tetracycline 45, 104
Third stage of labor 161, 162
Thyroid medicine 95
Toxemia 91, 121, 122, 123, 128, 135, 137, 205
    albumin in urine 121, 122
    avoidance 122
    blood pressure 121, 122, 123
    blurring of vision 121
    headache 121
    little urine 121
    pain 121
    swelling 121, 122
    symptoms 121
    water retention 121
Tranquilizers 62
    ransfusions, exchange 74
*Trichomoniasis* 102
Trimesters 31, 58
Triplets 126
Tubal pregnancy 117, 118, 119
    bathroom sign 118
    causes 117
    defective cilia 117
    diagnosis 118
    infection 117
    oversized egg 117
    pregnancy test 118
    recurrence 119
    surgery 119
    symptoms 118
Tuberculosis 131
Tumors 8

Twins 125, 126, 128, 169
    complications 128
    delivery 128
    nursing 169
    premature birth 128

**U**

Ultrasound 26, 125, 126, 129-132
    chromosomal damage 129
    complications 129
    retarded chromosomal growth 129
    uses 132
Umbilical cord 17, 22, 24, 128, 135, 182, 195
    blood vessels 24
    compression 128
    prolapse 128, 135, 182
Urinary tract infection 42, 132
Urination 7, 36, 91
    burning 91
    frequent 7
Urine
    albumin 205
    fetus' 17
    reduced amount 91
    specimen 42
Uterine bleeding 83
Uterine contractions 83
Uterus 48, 139, 162, 191
    massage 162
    tipped 191

**V**

Vacutage 111
Vagina 7, 8, 10, 62, 101, 118, 133, 155, 159, 162, 186, 188
Vaginal discharge 85, 99, 101, 190
    increase of 101
    irritation 101
    itching 101
    odor 101
    swelling 101
Vaginal exam 22
Vaginal infection 99-104
Varicose veins 115, 128, 206, 209
Veins 34, 206
Venereal disease, see *Sexually Transmitted Diseases*
Vernix 27
Vision 42, 91, 121
    blurring 121
    problems 91
Vitamins 49, 55, 60, 139
Vomiting, see *Nausea*

**W**

Walking 67
Water retention 48, 121
Water, sudden gush of 91
Weight gain 4, 48, 137, 139
    excessive 137, 139
Weight loss 53, 141, 194
Weight-control pills 62

**X**

X-ray 58, 125, 129-132, 152

**Y**

Yeast infection 104, 105